28 DAYS

OF

CHAIR YOGA

---

28 DAYS

OF

CHAIR EXERCISES

FOR WEIGHT LOSS

FOR SENIORS

Ottie Oz

Table of Contents

28 DAYS OF CHAIR YOGA

Introduction 9

How Will You Benefit from This Book? 11

Chair Yoga Misconceptions 13

How to Use This Book 15

Considerations 18

Getting Ready for Chair Yoga 21

Day 1: Neck, Shoulder, Arms, and Upper Back Relief 24

Day 2: Glutes, Lower Back, and Knees Strengthening 29

Day 3: Feet, Ankles, Hamstrings, and Quadriceps Care 34

Day 4: Shoulder and Arms Mobility 39

Day 5: Hip Openers, Knees, Upper Back, and Pelvic Release . . .44

Day 6: Shoulder, Arms, and Wrist Exercises 50

Day 7: Lower Back, Hamstrings, and Neck Relaxation 55

Day 8: Hamstrings, Hip Openers, Quadriceps, and
Upper Back Flow 60

Day 9: Empowering Lower Back, Neck, Shoulders, Arms,
and Upper Back 65

Day 10: Abdominals, Hip Openers, Knees, Quadriceps, and
Upper Back Revitalization 70

Day 11: Upper Back, Hip, Pelvic, Shoulder, and Arm Harmony . . .76

Day 12: Psoas Release for Upper Back Comfort 82

Day 13: Abdominals, Feet and Ankles, Hips, and
Lower Back Wellness .87

Day 14: Hip Openers, Lower Back, and Neck Relief with
Core Activation. 92

Day 15: Hamstrings, Hips, Knees, and Quadriceps Care 97

Day 16: Feet and Ankles Renewal — Completing a
Balanced Journey. 103

Day 17: Holistic Balance — A Full Body Journey 108

Day 18: Nurturing Feet, Ankles, Hip Openers, and
Quadriceps 113

Day 19: Biceps Triceps, Abs, and Knees. 118

Day 20: Hip Openers, Psoas Muscle, Hamstrings,
Abs, and Lower Back Harmony. 123

Day 21: Gentle Restoration — Neck, Biceps, Hips, and Knees. . . 129

Day 22: Hamstrings, Abs, Knees, Shoulders, and
Gluteus Strength 134

Day 23: Comprehensive Renewal Routine 138

Day 24: Comprehensive Muscle Focus 143

Day 25: Muscle Activation. 149

Day 26: Sun Salutation on the Chair 154

Day 27: Joyful Joints 157

Day 28: Core Strengthening and Lower Body Care 163

Conclusion 181
You Could Be Key to Someone Else's Yoga Journey 183
References 196

28 DAYS OF CHAIR EXERCISES

Introduction 203

Being Active and Embracing Fitness at Any Age 205

Managing Weight Loss with Exercises and Savvy
Food Choices 210

Finding Your Why, Committing to New Routines,
And Achieving Your Fitness Goals 217

Understanding Chair Exercises and the Benefits Of Them . . .224
    Benefits of Front Raises 224
    Benefits of Lateral Raises 225
    Benefits of Overhead Presses, Back Presses, and Front Presses 225
    Benefits of Core Strengthening Exercises 225
    Benefits of Seated Cardio Exercises 226
    Benefits of Quadriceps Muscle Exercises 226
    Benefits of Modified Sumo Chair and Chair Squats 227

How to Use This Book and Frequently Asked Questions 228
    How to Use This Book 228
    Frequently Asked Questions 229

Room 232

Initiating Your Chair Exercise Journey: Correct Posture 233

Three Warm-Up and Cooldown Routines. 236
    Warm-Up One 238
    Warm-Up Two 241
    Warm-Up Three 243
    Cooldown Routine 246

Day 1 249
Day 2 252
Day 3 255

Day 4 257

Day 5 260

Day 6 262

Day 7 265

Day 8 268

Day 9 270

Day 10 273

Day 11. 276

Day 12 279

Day 13. 282

Day 14. 284

Day 15. 288

Day 16. 291

Day 17. 294

Day 18. 297

Day 19. 299

Day 20 302

Day 21. 306

Day 22 309

Day 23 311

Day 24 314

Day 25 316

Day 26 320

Day 27 323

Day 28 325

Conclusion 328

You Could Be Key to Someone Else's Yoga Journey 329

References 333

Build Strength, Boost Flexibility,
and Increase Balance
in Just 10 Minutes a Day

28 DAYS

OF

CHAIR YOGA

FOR SENIORS

Ottie Oz

A Gift to Our Readers

I'm thrilled to include a special gift for our readers *15 Guided Meditations*.

These 15 guided voice meditations provide a unique opportunity to enhance your practice. They're designed to be accessible and convenient for your busy lifestyle.

Unlock the power and experience the countless benefits they offer.

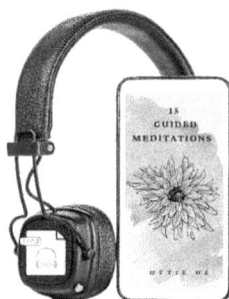

Elevate your practice, enhance your well-being, and embrace the serenity that awaits you.

Scan QR code

Introduction

"Yoga is not about touching your toes.
It is what you learn on the way down."

– Jigar Gor

This transformative guide is created to strengthen your body, increase your mobility, and improve your overall well-being. In 28 days, these routines will empower you to become stronger, leaner, and more balanced—all in less than 10 minutes daily. You will find 28 daily chair yoga routines designed to work on different body parts to help you become stronger and increase your mobility.

Whether you're new to yoga or have been practicing for years, this book is designed with the more mature population in mind. So grab a chair and get ready to discover the incredible benefits of *Chair Yoga for Seniors!*

Staying active becomes even more crucial as we age. Our bodies naturally start to lose muscle mass and bone density. Regular exercise helps maintain strength in our muscles and bones, reducing the risk of falls and fractures. Maintaining our physical fitness and overall health becomes increasingly important. But that doesn't mean we have to surrender to the challenges of time. Instead, we can adapt and discover new ways to nurture our bodies and minds. Chair yoga is one such pathway—a gentle, accessible, and incredibly effective practice tailor-made for people with reduced mobility due to different health conditions. No matter your age, various health conditions can affect you earlier in life, and not all, even young people, can exercise lying on the floor.

Regarding staying active and healthy, chair yoga or any other chair exercises are a game-changer. This gentle exercise offers numerous benefits that can enhance your overall well-being. Chair yoga helps improve flexibility and range of motion. The gentle stretches in seated positions target key muscle groups, helping increase joint mobility and relieve stiffness.

Not only does chair yoga boost physical health, but it also promotes mental wellness. Regular chair yoga sessions help reduce stress levels and improve relaxation. Focusing on deep breathing techniques aids in calming the mind, promoting mindfulness, and reducing anxiety.

Chair yoga is an inclusive practice accommodating individuals with various physical abilities or limitations. Incorporating chair yoga into your routine can enhance balance and stability—a crucial aspect for seniors—reducing the chances of falls or accidents.

It also provides numerous physical, mental, and emotional benefits, such as improved balance, flexibility, and muscle strength, and reduces stressful health by increasing blood circulation and lowering blood pressure.

Engaging in regular physical activity is not only beneficial for the body but also for mental health. In addition to improving memory and concentration, endorphins that boost mood and reduce stress are released when exercising.

Chair yoga provides a gentle yet effective way for anyone to incorporate movement into their daily routine. This form of yoga adapts traditional poses to be performed while seated or using a chair for support.

How Will You Benefit from This Book?

With this book as your guide, you can expect clear instructions accompanied by illustrations for each exercise. In this *28 Days of Chair Yoga*, you will experience many benefits that can significantly enhance your overall well-being. Incorporating movements and stretches into your daily routine will improve your physical health and nurture your mental and emotional wellness. Don't underestimate the power of this modified practice—it can work wonders for your body and mind!

With each day's practice, you'll notice increased flexibility in your muscles and joints. It may also help reduce joint, head, and back pains. The gentle stretching exercise routines in the book will help to alleviate stiffness and promote a better range of motion. This can be especially beneficial for those with limited mobility or who struggle with arthritis or other conditions.

Chair yoga is also an excellent way to improve balance and stability. Maintaining our equilibrium becomes increasingly important as we age to prevent falls and injuries. The various poses in this book target specific muscle groups that support balance, helping to strengthen them over time.

Furthermore, regular chair yoga sessions promote better circulation throughout the body. Moving the body gently while seated improves blood flow, providing essential nutrients to all organs and tissues. This enhanced circulation can lead to improved energy levels and reduced fatigue.

But it's not just physical benefits that make chair yoga so valuable; it also significantly impacts mental well-being. Practicing mindfulness through focused breathing exercises helps calm the mind and reduce stress. It provides an opportunity for relaxation amidst the hustle of everyday life.

With its easy-to-follow routines specifically designed for older adults, it offers immense value both physically and emotionally.

Age should never hinder us from living our best lives! Embrace the benefits of chair yoga and experience a renewed sense of vitality, strength, and inner peace.

Exercise also boosts mental health by reducing symptoms of anxiety and depression while promoting cognitive function. Staying active keeps our minds sharp and improves memory recall.

Another reason why exercise is vital for seniors is its ability to increase mobility and independence. Strong muscles support joint function, making everyday tasks easier to perform without assistance.

Furthermore, regular exercise promotes better sleep patterns, which is crucial for overall health maintenance.

Chair Yoga Misconceptions

Many misconceptions about chair yoga are circulating, and a few of them are present here.

It's Too Easy: One of the common misconceptions is that chair yoga may not provide a challenging workout compared to other forms of exercise. However, this couldn't be further from the truth! Chair Yoga can help build core strength, enhance muscle tone, and boost overall stamina by engaging in controlled movements and focusing on proper breathing techniques. Some people mistakenly believe that chair yoga is not challenging enough to provide real health benefits. While gentle and accessible, chair yoga can be adapted to different fitness levels, and its effectiveness should not be underestimated. The practice can be demanding, depending on the poses and exercises' intensity.

Another incredible aspect of chair yoga is its ability to promote relaxation and reduce stress. Through guided meditation and mindful breathing exercises incorporated into the practice, participants experience improved mental clarity, reduced anxiety, and enhanced emotional well-being.

It's Only for Seniors: While chair yoga is excellent for seniors due to its accessibility and focus on gentle movements, it's not exclusive to this demographic. Chair yoga can benefit people of all ages and fitness levels. Athletes, office workers, and those recovering from injuries or surgery can find value in chair yoga's adaptability.

It's Not a "Real" Form of Yoga: Some believe chair yoga is not authentic because it adapts traditional yoga poses for seated practice. However, chair yoga incorporates the fundamental principles of yoga, including mindfulness, breathing techniques, and the mind-body connection. It's a legitimate and effective form of yoga.

Boring: In reality, chair yoga can be enjoyable and mentally stimulating. It offers opportunities for self-reflection, relaxation, and the development of mindfulness skills. Many practitioners find it a rewarding and calming practice.

And these are just some of them. So, if you're wondering whether chair yoga works, try it yourself! You'll soon discover how this accessible exercise can transform physical health while promoting inner peace and harmony. Give it a chance; remember that to see the improvement, you need time.

So stick to the program and let me know what you think.

Moreover, regular practice of chair yoga has been shown to boost mental well-being by reducing stress levels. It provides an opportunity for relaxation through deep breathing techniques.

How to Use This Book

"Yoga reminds me that everything is connected,
so we must live, act, and breathe with awareness."
— Adrien Mishler

Regardless of whether you decide to follow this program or not and which page you will start from, it's recommended to read this chapter and what you need to start your journey.

28 Days Chair Yoga Program is great for:

- Beginners who want to start practicing chair yoga
- People with reduced mobility
- People who are looking for low-impact exercise but still want to have a workout
- Individuals who are recovering from surgeries or injuries
- Sedentary individuals who want to offset the negative effects of prolonged sitting
- Yoga teachers looking for new ideas and ways to improve routines for their students

If this is something you think is for you, then keep exploring.

This book has 28 sequences and three bonus ones.

Each day, you will perform different sequences. They all have descriptions of what the routine is focused on. The benefit of it is that you can choose which one you prefer to do or simply follow the program.

If a certain day's routine looks challenging or you feel like your joints need attention on that day, then you can switch the days you're working on.

Also, if you feel that you want a longer session, you can always do an extra day or add one of the bonus sequences. Also, you can repeat the same routine twice.

Find what feels good and make this journey your own.

Never push or continue doing poses if you feel pain. This is your body, and only you know what feels right for it. Stop and listen. It's a journey of respect, discovering your potential, and accepting your limits. Some days, we're strong, and some days, we need to be quiet. Do what feels good. Listen to your body and heart. Be who you are when no one is watching.

All 28 routines have pictures at the back of the book. Once you become comfortable and know how to perform the poses, you can use only pictures as your guide.

Each routine includes light warm-up moves. Before you start the routine, sit in the mountain pose position and gather your thoughts—concentrate on your breath and coordinate your breath with the movement. Finish the routine as well in a mountain pose, savoring the fruit of your practice. When you practice, once you're sitting in a mountain pose position, remember a few things to observe when practicing:

Don't lift your shoulders to your ears unless you're doing shoulder shrugs.

Think that you have a lot of space between your earlobes and shoulders; your neck is nice and tall. Your head is aligned above your heart. You sit relaxed yet with your core engaged and your spine straight. Try to do your body's best. Always think about your breath—don't hold it. It must flow at your pace, in and out.

Considerations

Please read before you proceed with the chair yoga routines.

If you are concerned about injuring yourself by practicing chair yoga, the best action is to talk to your doctor or physical therapist. Show them the chair yoga routines you plan to practice and ask them to recommend postures suitable for your health condition.

It's important to remember that yogic postures are eased into slowly, and there is a heightened focus on the body. Try one of the variations if you struggle to ease into an asana. If none of the variations work, skip that asana and move on to the next. You should never be in pain while practicing. If you feel or experience any pain, do not push yourself further.

Another important aspect of being comfortable while in asanas is remembering to breathe. It would be best if you were not holding your breath while in an asana unless directed to do so—and even when required to do so, it should never be longer than a couple of seconds. This is why it would be beneficial to practice breathing exercises every day.

Important things to remember while practicing chair yoga (or yoga of any kind):

- Consistency is the key to achieving your goals. Practice regularly. You will not acquire any results by practicing once every other week.
- You don't have to have the perfect form. Follow the directions to the best of your ability and only to a point where you are comfortable.

- Yoga is not a competition or a race. Work at your own pace and use the best variations for you.

- Pay attention to your head and neck alignment to avoid pain.

- Sit toward the front edge of the chair with your feet flat on the floor, hip-width apart. This position provides stability and allows for better alignment during poses.

- Work on coordinating breath and movement. Listen to your body. You can keep your knees together or apart. Keep arms on your thighs with palms up or down. There is no right or wrong; there is you and what feels good to you.

- Sit up straight with your spine aligned and shoulders relaxed. Proper posture is essential for safe and effective chair yoga.

- Incorporate mindful breathing throughout your practice. Deep, rhythmic breathing can help you relax and enhance your focus on each pose.

- Drink water before and after your practice to stay hydrated, especially if your session is more prolonged or intense.

- There are recommendations for how many breaths to hold the pose. However, if you want to reduce or add more breaths to your poses—feel free to do so. Don't feel bad if you cannot hold a pose for three breaths. It's not a competition. This is your journey. Holding the position for three breaths might be a challenge initially, but with 20 days of practice, you could comfortably sustain the pose for four breaths. Your body will naturally adapt, desiring to linger in the position for an extended duration.

- Those with **spinal disc problems** or **glaucoma** should take special care to choose postures without twists or inversions. NEVER force yourself into a twisted position, or any position for that matter, using your hands and forcing yourself. When performing forward bending, move from the hip joint without rounding your back. Avoid bouncing and impact.

- Chair yoga is not just about physical movement; it is also about mindfulness and relaxation. Stay present and focus on your breath and sensations throughout the practice.
- Don't let your ego get in the way—listen to your BODY.
- It is better not to have a big meal before practicing chair yoga.

We all have different bodies, and their abilities are different. Some days you will feel better, some days not, and it's OK. There is that hype that every day should be perfect; if it's not, then it's a failure. And then we're getting upset and disappointed with ourselves that we failed. We have failed to have a good day! This is just wild! We must accept that we have bad, mediocre, sound, and perfect days. And when it's a 'bad' day, we take it, move on, and do our best to be the best versions of ourselves. We cannot always be happy, content, and on top of the world, constantly feeling the winners. We don't always feel great physically; we ache and hurt. It's not about having a perfect day; it's about accepting the things that we cannot change and moving on. It's about having the wisdom to identify what we can change and the strength to change it.

If you haven't exercised in years, you cannot expect your body to perform at top-notch ability. However, you can expect your body to get there. Chair yoga is not a competition, and it's not about twisting yourself into a pretzel.

It's about your journey. It's about what you will discover.

Getting Ready for Chair Yoga

An Attitude

Sometimes, people, including myself, lose their motivation or their 'why.' Think of your own; why have you decided to do this program? Once you have your why, then remember it when you feel down or are unwilling to do a routine. Remember that the most challenging thing is to show up for your practice. Once you're on the chair—the hard part is done.

Consistency is key. Regular chair yoga practice can improve your balance and flexibility over time. Aim for short, frequent sessions rather than occasional long ones.

Clothing

You don't need fancy yoga clothing. Don't use this as an excuse not to start the program. You should wear something comfortable that will allow you to move around easily. Sometimes, I do my short morning routines in my pajamas because no one is watching, and I feel like it!

Yoga Mat

You don't necessarily need a yoga mat. However, often, people put a yoga mat under the chair to prevent it from sliding. Also, if you prefer to exercise bare feet, it helps prevent friction.

Chair

You need a sturdy chair with no arms. The absence of arms allows for greater flexibility in movement, and the key is to select a chair that remains steadfast throughout your yoga routine, providing stability without shifting or moving. Choose any regular sturdy chair for exercises; steer clear of folding chairs or those with wheels.

Socks or No Socks?

It's your preference. You can exercise bare feet. If you choose to wear socks, make sure they have a grip on their soles.

Room

You can exercise in any room or use an outside space.

If this is an option, I prefer to open the windows to feel the fresh air getting in. But this is only my preference. This is your practice, your choice.

Ensure you have enough free space around you—no sharp objects, corners, or furniture nearby. The room doesn't have to be furniture-free. However, a tidy space can help create a calming atmosphere for your practice.

Now, let's transition into the practical part of this program. These chair yoga routines enhance your flexibility, balance, and overall well-being. As you go through these exercises, remember to honor your body's limitations and make sure to progress at a comfortable pace. Let's get started to kickstart your chair yoga practice!

Type the following into your browser to access a complete list of chair yoga demonstrations. Please note that the link is **_case sensitive,_** so if you mistype it, it will not work.

https://www.youtube.com/@ZenflowHub/playlists

The videos are designed to assist you in performing the chair yoga poses detailed in this book. They serve as a valuable resource for checking your form or for additional clarification on the exercise techniques. The demonstrations include all exercises covered in the book. There are 28 videos, one for each day. They're silent videos as their purpose is to demonstrate the poses if you're in doubt or prefer to watch them first. They're designed as a secondary resource, providing a little visual help to supplement the book.

NECK, SHOULDER, ARMS, AND UPPER BACK RELIEF

This chair yoga routine provides targeted relief for your neck, shoulders, arms, and upper back. Throughout the sequence, you'll engage in gentle movements that focus on loosening tension in these key muscle groups. By incorporating stretches and poses specifically tailored for the upper body, you'll experience improved flexibility and circulation, promoting relaxation, reducing discomfort, and building strength.

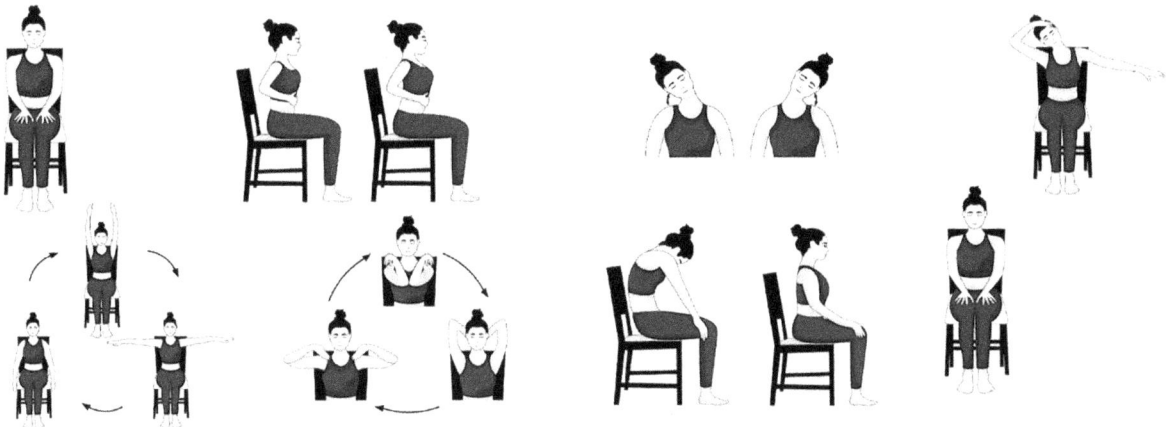

Mountain Pose

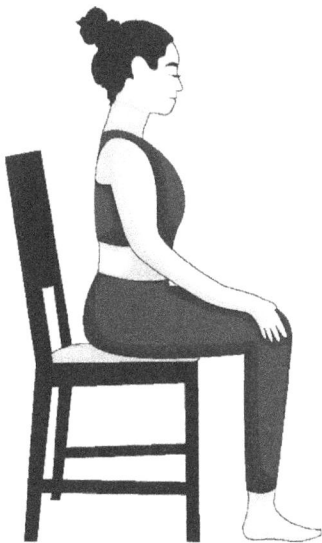

Find a comfortable seated position in the center of the chair, leaving some space between the back of the chair and your back. Rock back and forth until you locate your sit bones. Keep your feet hip-distance apart and flat on the floor. If you prefer, bring your knees together. Take a few deep breaths to center yourself and bring your awareness to the present moment. Begin by gently closing your eyes or softening your gaze. Let go of any distractions and allow your mind to settle. Bring your attention to your breath. Feel the rise and fall of your abdomen with each inhale and exhale. Notice how it feels as it flows in and out of your nose. Follow the breath with your attention, noticing the coolness of the inhale and the warmth of the exhale. Stay for ten breaths, and when ready, move on to the next exercise.

Seated Pelvic Tilt Tuck

Place feet firmly on the floor in mountain pose, arms resting on your knees, and spine erect. Place your hands on top of the pelvis crest to feel the movement. This is a slight movement, just tilting the tailbone back and forth.

Inhale as you tilt the pelvis forward. Exhale as you tilt the pelvis backward. Repeat for six to eight cycles.

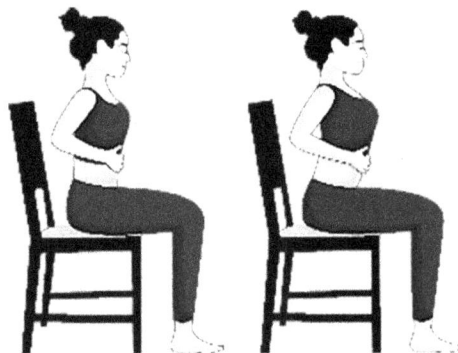

Chair Neck Rolls

Take a couple of deep breaths. Inhale, move your ear toward the right shoulder, and exhale. Make sure that the neck is long, and the shoulders are relaxed and away from the ears. On the inhale, come back to the center, exhale, and pause before switching sides. Repeat on another side, three to five times on both sides.

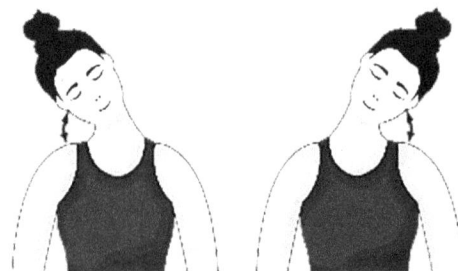

Chair Neck Stretch

Sit comfortably in the chair, knees stacked over ankles at 90 degrees. Exhale, tilting head right, right hand on left ear, and left arm extended. Inhale, return to center. Exhale, tilt head left, left hand on right ear, and right arm extended. Repeat two more times on both sides.

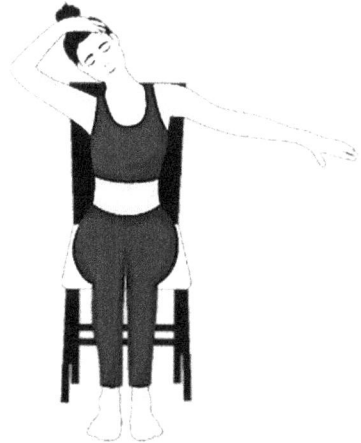

Chair Mountain Pose Sweeping Arms Flow

Sit in a mountain pose. Inhale, reaching the arms up, palms facing each other above your head. Exhale and slowly release them down, palms facing down. Inhale, reaching the arms up; exhale with palms facing down. Repeat the sequence for another five times.

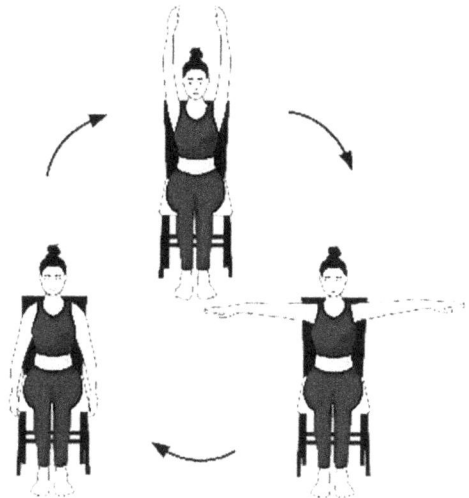

Shoulder Socket Rotation

Sit up tall with your back straight. Bring the fingertips to rest on the shoulders.

On the inhale, begin to move the bent elbows from the center, moving upward.

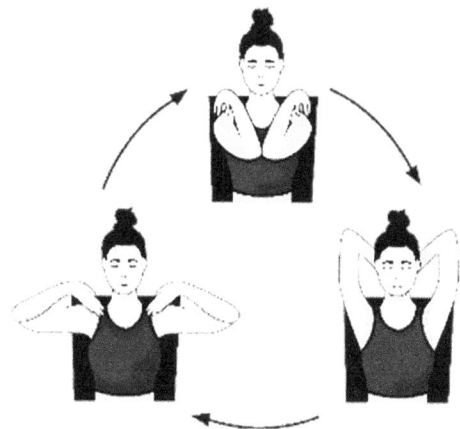

Move them in a circular movement from the center about six times. Repeat the opposite direction another six times. Watch your breath, and work on coordinating the action with your breath at your own pace.

Chair Cat-Cow Pose

Place your arms on your knees. As you inhale, expand your chest, allowing your head and chin to tilt slightly back. On the exhale, round your spine by curling your chest inward. Ensure your shoulders are relaxed and be aware of the space between your shoulders and earlobes. Practice coordinating your breath with the movement, moving at a comfortable pace. Repeat five to eight times.

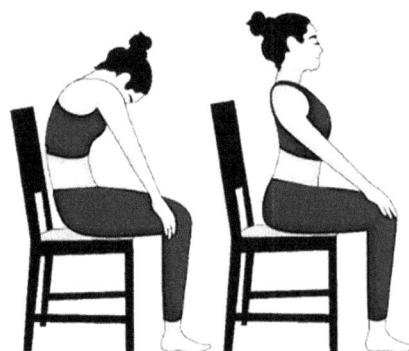

Mountain Pose

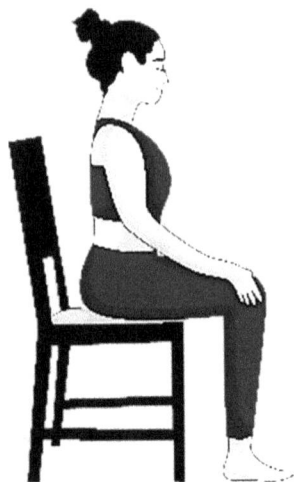

Find a comfortable seated position in the center of the chair, leaving some space between the back of the chair and your back. Take a few deep breaths and say thanks. You've done well.

Day 2

GLUTES, LOWER BACK, AND KNEES STRENGTHENING

Today, you'll engage in a series of movements designed to strengthen and support the glutes, lower back, knees, shoulders, and arms. Focusing on these muscle groups will enhance overall stability and mobility. The routine incorporates poses and stretches that target the glutes and lower back, promoting a stronger core and reduced lower back discomfort.

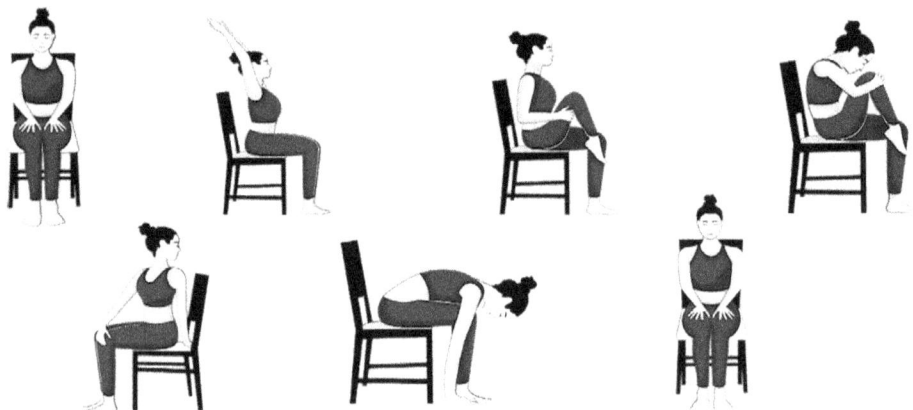

Mountain Pose

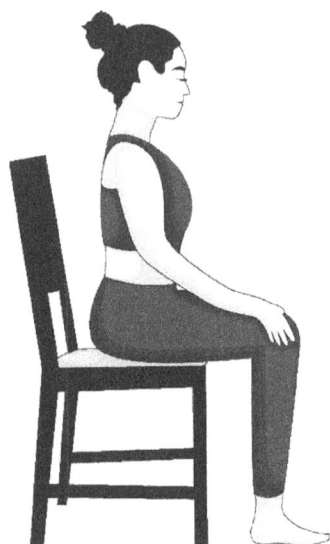

It's your Day 2 when you have shown up for your practice. The hardest part is done. Take a few deep breaths, feel like the air travels into your lungs, and on the exhale, the warm air comes out. Today, you will learn *Right Nostril Breathing Variation Close Up*. This breath practice of the right nostril helps to revitalize the body. It increases the efficiency of the digestive system and also boosts the nervous system, especially the sympathetic nervous system. Close the left nostril with the little finger and ring finger, and breathe in and out through the right. Avoid if blood pressure is high. Do two rounds four times each.

Hands Up Chair

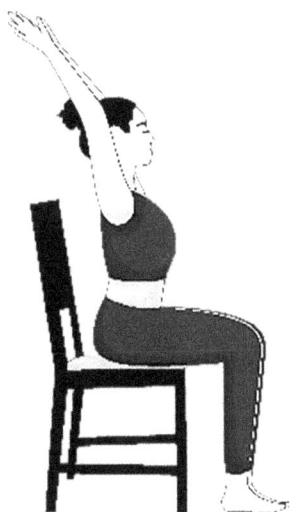

Gently roll your shoulders back, feel your core muscles engaged, and raise your arms above your head on the inhale. Keep shoulders relaxed and away from your ears. Keep the palms facing and touching each other. If not, leave some distance between them; imagine that you're holding a big ball above your head.

If keeping both arms above your head is difficult, bend them slightly through the elbows. Or practice one arm at a time. Keep your arms above your head for a few cycles of breath. Raise your chin slightly, but do not drop your head back. On the exhale, lower your arms. Repeat this cycle two to three times, holding for two to three breaths.

Seated Low Lunge Variation Chair

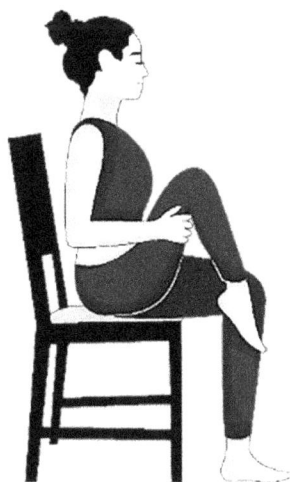

Observe your breath and move from the mountain pose; bend your right knee toward your chest on the inhale. Place your arms behind your thigh and hold the right thigh with your hands while flexing the knee. Try to keep your torso straight, and don't hold your breath.

If you need, lean back for support. Feel the stretch at the hips, lower back, hamstrings, knee, and ankle. Stay in the pose for about three to six breaths. Switch sides.

Knee Head Down Chair

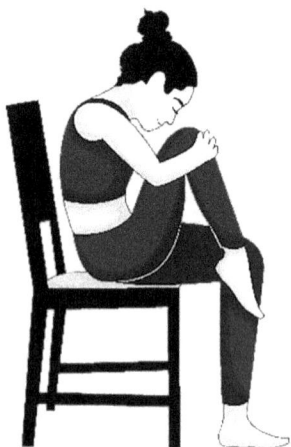

Releasing from the previous pose, inhale, and while you exhale, press the thighs closer to you while you bring the face toward the knee, flexing the neck. Press the thighs, and rest the nose on the knee in the Knee Head Down Chair pose for about three to six breaths. Resting the back completely, make sure you get a grip on the hips and the foot on the floor to avoid slipping from the chair. Repeat the move with the opposite leg.

Chair Seated Twists

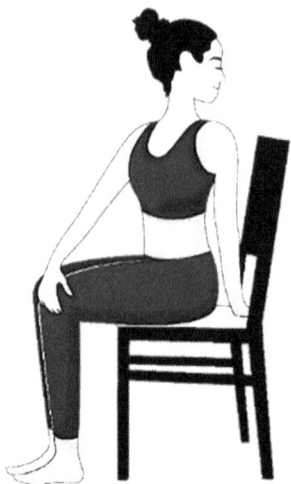

Make sure you're not leaning on the back of the chair. Rock forward and back; find your sit bones. Sit tall with feet touching the floor and knees hip-width apart.

Inhale and place your arms over your head—lift and lengthen.

With the exhalation, twist left from the base of the spine. Your ribcage, shoulders, neck, and eyes go to the left, but the hips remain on the chair. The right hand goes to the left knee, and the left hand is behind the left hip or on the back of the chair. Stay in the position for three deep breaths. Repeat the opposite side, twice each side.

Seated Forward Fold Pose on Chair

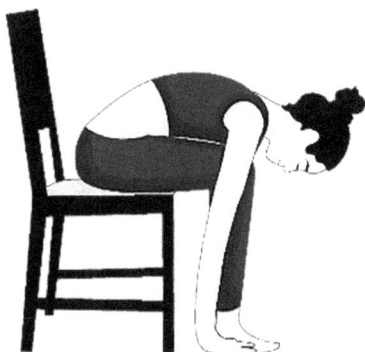

While seated in the mountain pose chair, breathe in deep a few times to relax and extend the spine. Exhaling, bring your arms down toward your feet, with the torso resting on the thighs and chin close to the knees. Stretching the shoulders, place your palms flat on the floor, and remain here for four breaths. As you exhale, push closer into the thighs and abdomen, stretching farther each time. To release, inhale, look up first, then raise your arms before coming back to sit. Remain in the pose for two breaths or till you feel comfortable.

Mountain Pose

Sit for a while, taking deep breaths. Soften your gaze or close your eyes completely. Scan your body for how it feels. Do you feel any tension? Direct your attention to your hands. Begin to move them mindfully, exploring different gestures and motions. Observe the sensations in your fingers, palms, and wrists as you move. Stay present in the experience of this movement. Feel the rise and fall of your abdomen with each inhale and exhale. Complete practice when you feel ready to move on with your daily tasks.

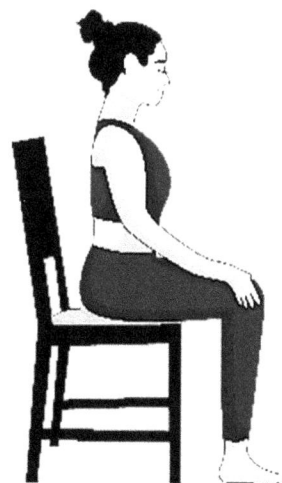

FEET, ANKLES, HAMSTRINGS, AND QUADRICEPS CARE

Dedicate today's chair yoga routine to the well-being of your feet, ankles, hamstrings, and quadriceps. This sequence focuses on providing gentle yet effective stretches and movements to support these crucial muscle groups. You'll improve flexibility, balance, and overall foot health by targeting the feet and ankles. The stretches for hamstrings and quadriceps help maintain proper leg muscle function, allowing for better mobility and reduced tightness.

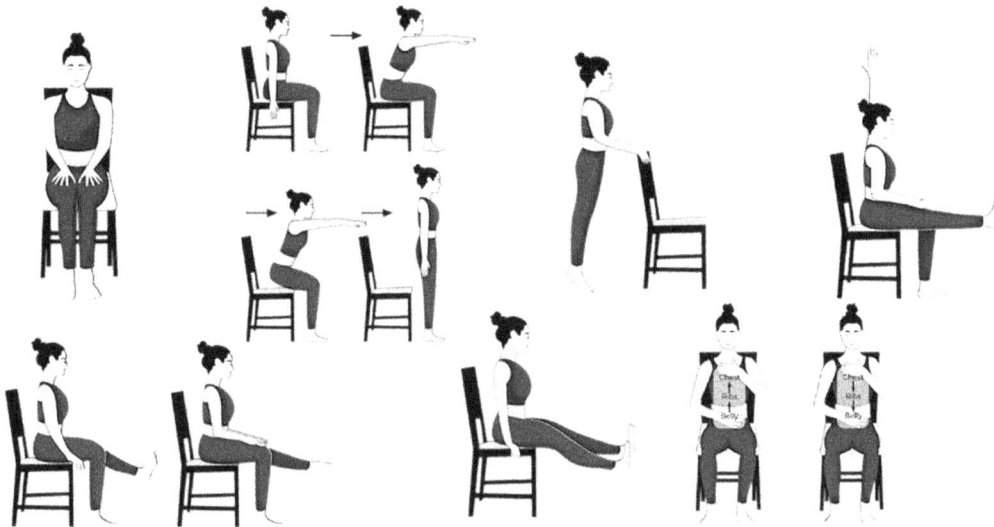

Chair Mountain Pose Stand-Up Flow

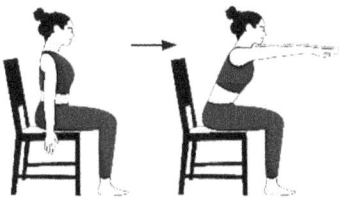

Start in a mountain pose. Feel the rise and fall of your abdomen with each inhale and exhale. Do five rounds, and feel the ground under your feet. Move your toes and feel each of them.

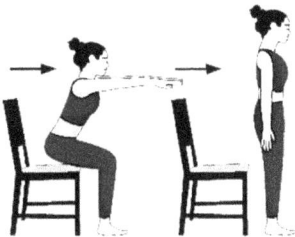

The spine is nice and tall, shoulders rolled back. Reach your arms forward to help you lift your hips off the chair. Hold this position for a couple of breaths; if not, stand up. Feel the ground under your feet. Sit back down with your arms next to you. Repeat five more times.

Heel Raises

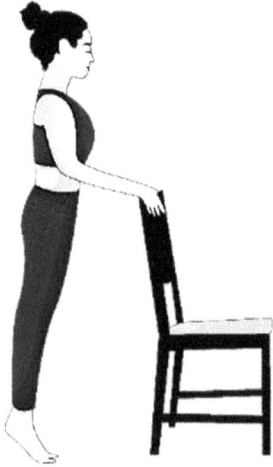

Use the chair's support when attempting heel raises if balance poses a challenge. If this is not an option, then do heel raises when sitting down in a mountain pose.

As you inhale, elevate your body, finding equilibrium on your toes, experiencing the sole's gentle stretch. This sensation extends from the hips, emphasizing a seamless connection to the leg stretch as you gradually rise. Maintain this posture for three to six breaths, then release and repeat. If this is too challenging, you can go up and down, as this is also a great way to stretch your feet.

Easy Pose Chair One Leg Opposite Arm Raised

Sit nice and tall, away from the chair back.

Engage your core, and pull the belly button toward the spine.

Inhale and raise the right leg and left arm. Hold for a few breaths.

Feel how your leg is activated. Lower the leg or bend through the knee if it's too challenging. Remember to breathe and coordinate movement with breath. Release to the ground after a couple of breaths. Repeat two to three times for each side.

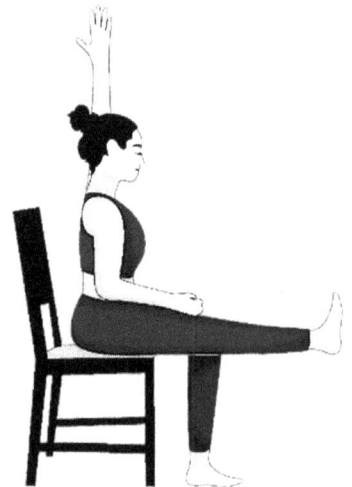

Chair Flexing Foot Pose

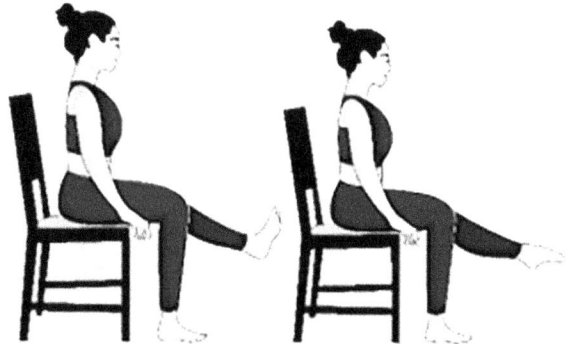

Lift your right leg, and point the toes away from you. As you inhale, lift your toes toward your face and press the heel away. Exhale, and point your toes outward. Repeat this sequence five times before switching to the other leg.

Staff Pose Chair

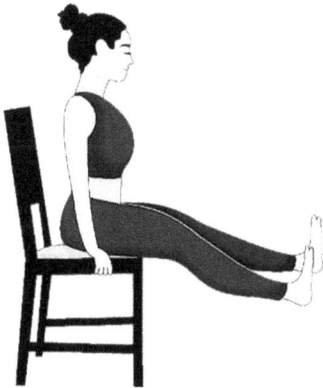

Sit upright with a straight spine and hold onto the sides of the chair seat with both hands. Engage your lower abdomen, and lift both legs simultaneously as you inhale. Keep your legs straight and parallel to the ground, flexing your feet upward. Wiggle your toes to keep your legs active, and if comfortable, hold this position for three breaths. If you cannot lift both legs simultaneously, try to alternate them. As you exhale, gently lower your legs back to the ground and return to a neutral seated position. Repeat it three times, resting in between.

Three-Part Breathing

Inhale

Exhale

To end the routine, let's practice a breathing exercise.

As you begin, you may place your hands on different body parts to feel the air expanding and contracting the area. Begin by inhaling air into your belly, allowing it to expand with each breath in and flatten with each exhale. Take your time to get comfortable with this motion.

Next, take a deep belly breath, and when your belly is expanded, draw in another small breath, and focus it into your lower chest. Place your hand on your lower chest to feel it expand.

When exhaling, first release the air from your chest, then from your belly, allowing both to deflate completely. Practice this until you feel comfortable with the movement.

Now, breathe into your belly, then into your lower chest, and finally, draw in one last breath to fill the upper chest, expanding it up to the collarbone. Feel your entire chest fully expand. When exhaling, start by releasing the air from your upper chest, then from your lower chest, and finally from your belly. Let each part deflate completely before moving on to the next.

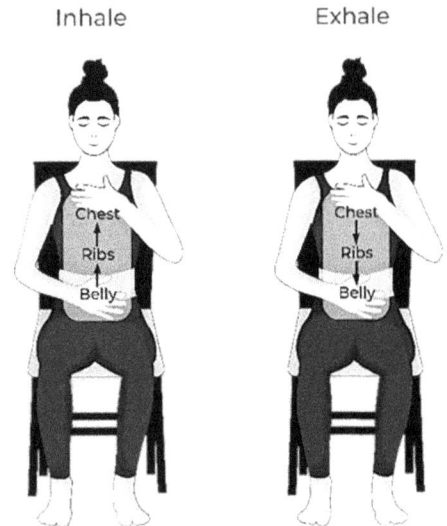

Day 4

SHOULDER AND ARMS MOBILITY

Today's chair yoga routine is dedicated to enhancing shoulder and arm mobility. Through gentle movements and stretches, you'll engage in exercises specifically designed to improve flexibility and strength in these crucial upper body areas. Focusing on the shoulders and arms will promote better posture, alleviate tension, and increase the overall range of motion. Regular practice will contribute to a more comfortable and functional upper body, allowing you to perform daily activities more efficiently. As you dedicate this time to your shoulder and arm well-being, you invest in your overall physical comfort and vitality.

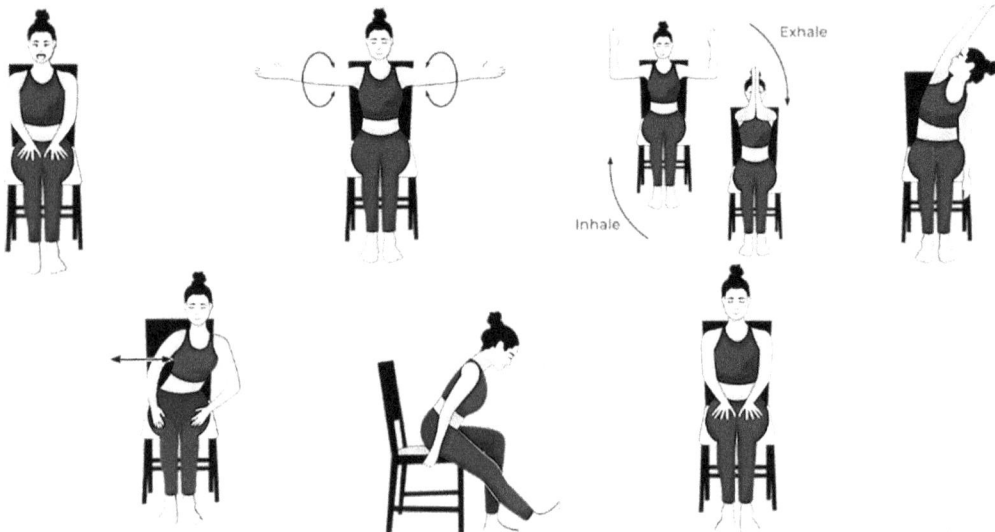

Lion's Breath (Simhasana)

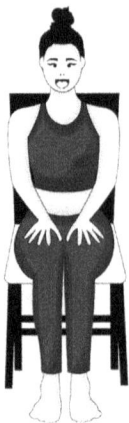

Sit comfortably on the chair and maintain a straight spine. You can lean on your chair backrest—as long as you sit tall with your shoulders lowered.

Unbend your arms and stretch out your fingers. This is to imitate a lion's claws. Inhale through the nostrils, then exhale with a loud "ha" from the mouth, extending your tongue as close to the chin as you can. While breathing out, focus on the middle of your forehead or the end of your nose. Fill up with breath, and go back to neutral facial expression. Repeat four to six times.

Arms to Side Rotations Chair

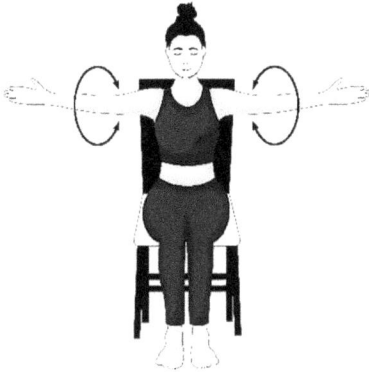

Raise your arms and spread them to the sides parallel to the floor, making a nice T. Breathe in and start making small circles with your wrists in one direction. After a couple of breaths, make a few circles in the opposite direction.

Start making small circles with your arms and slowly increase the motion, making them bigger, and then again, start rotating your arms in the opposite direction, making the circles small until you find stillness.

Seated Cactus Arms Flow Chair

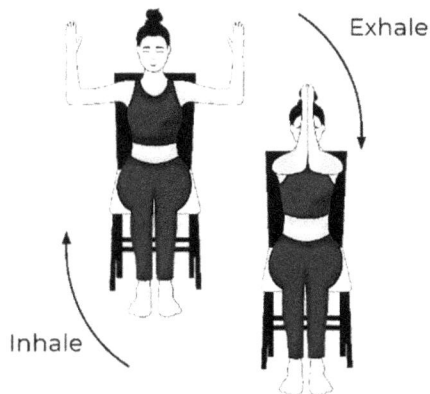

Cactus arms, elbows in line with shoulders, wrists stacked over elbows. Spread the fingers and point them up. Breathe in, and bring your arms to the side with your elbows bent as pictured. Take a deep breath, lift through the chest, and squeeze the shoulder blades together. Listen to your body. As you exhale, bring your elbows, forearms, and hands together. Inhale, open your arms into a cactus position, and squeeze your shoulder blades together. Repeat the flow three to five times. Work on coordinating the flow with the breath.

Chair Seated Side Stretch Pose

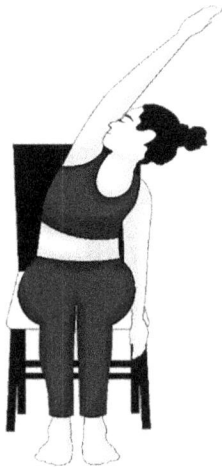

Sit upright. Place the hands on either side of the seat or your lap. Roll your shoulders down the back. Inhale and, pulling in the core, sweep the right arm above the head, creating a lateral bend on the left-hand side. Exhale into the stretch. Allow your chest and head to tilt to the left. Stay in this pose for three breaths. On the inhale, return to the center. Repeat the same with the left side.

You can choose to stay on one side for two to three breaths before switching to the other side, or you may choose to move dynamically between one side and the other on the breath. Do what feels best for your body.

Chair Torso Circles

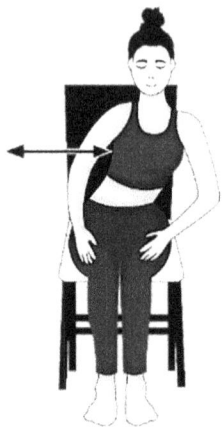

Feel your sit bones firmly grounded to the chair. Inhale, rolling your ribs forward.

Exhale and round your back, ensuring only the torso moves while your legs stay grounded. Draw circles, adjust the size as needed, and listen to your body.

Repeat this movement three to five times at your own breath pace. Change direction and repeat the process.

Half Seated Forward Bend Pose Chair

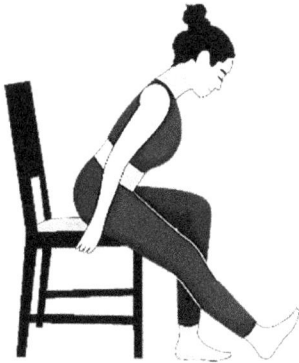

While seated on the chair, move your thighs forward and extend your right leg, placing the foot out and resting it on the heels. Point your toes upward and press the heels firmly to stretch the sole of your foot. Take a moment to feel the sensation of the stretch in the inner sole, and remain in this position, breathing deeply for about three to six breaths. Focus on extending the quads, hamstrings, and calves, feeling release and relaxation in those areas.

Now, repeat the same sequence with the other leg. Pay attention to the leg with more issues and try to hold that stretch a bit longer. You can repeat this stretching process multiple times to work on the tendons and tissues around the plantar fascia (ligament). After completing both legs, take a moment to relax and settle into your seated position.

Day 5

HIP OPENERS, KNEES, UPPER BACK, AND PELVIC RELEASE

Today's practice offers a comprehensive approach to nurturing multiple muscle groups. You'll focus on hip openers, external rotation, knees, shoulders, arms, upper back, and pelvic release. Gentle poses and stretches promote flexibility and relieve tension in these diverse areas. Hip openers and external rotation exercises improve hip mobility, while knee-focused movements support joint health and flexibility. The routine also addresses shoulder, arm, and upper back comfort, reducing muscle tightness and promoting relaxation.

Additionally, pelvic release poses benefit your core and lower back, enhancing overall posture and stability. By engaging in this well-rounded practice, you'll experience improved mobility, reduced discomfort, and enhanced body awareness. Take time to care for these interconnected muscle groups, fostering a sense of balance and harmony throughout your body.

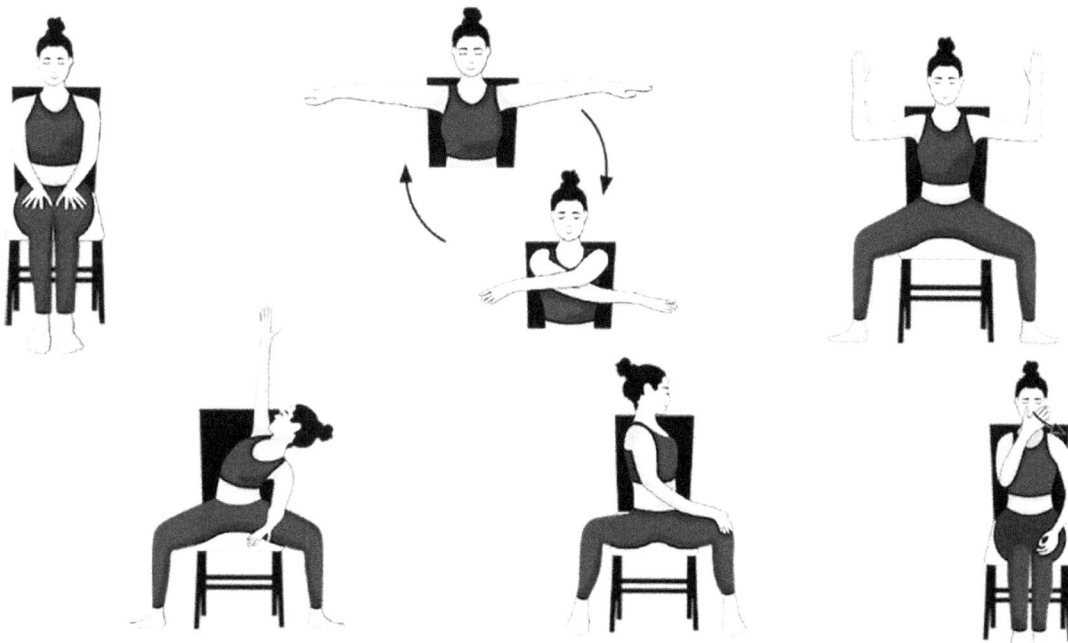

Let's begin in a mountain pose with your arms pressed against your chest.

Take a few deep breaths and become aware of your surroundings. Breathe in, identify the smell, listen carefully, and identify what you can hear around you. Now, shift your focus to your body. Start from your toes, and slowly scan your way up, paying attention to any sensations, tensions, or areas of tightness that you may feel. Take a few moments to breathe into those areas and release any tension or discomfort. When ready—move on to the next step.

Arms Swing Pose Flow Close Up

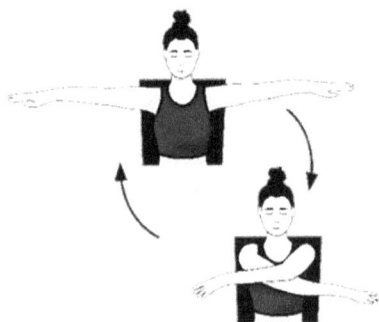

Exercises like arm swings warm up and stretch the shoulders, arms, chest, and upper back, preparing the muscles, tendons, and joints for other poses. Raise your arms sideways, parallel to the floor. Allow your arms to swing forward, hands crossing over each other. Swing arms back, then forward again, alternating which hand swings over the top of the other. This movement may not be in time with your breath, and that is okay. Continue the movement for three to five breaths. You can repeat it twice.

Goddess Pose on Chair

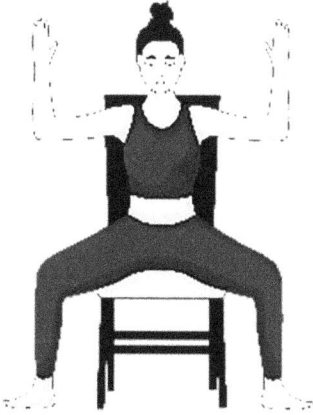

Sit comfortably in the middle of the chair, ensuring there is some space between your back and the backrest. Open your legs wide, keeping your knees aligned over your ankles with your toes slightly turned out. Press through your sit bones and feel grounded through all four corners of your feet. Lengthen your spine and maintain an upright posture. Extend your arms and bend at the elbows, creating a cactus pose with palms facing forward. Slightly squeeze your shoulder blades together. Lift your chest up and outward, feeling the engagement of your shoulder blades and the opening of your heart. To maintain an active stance, gently press through your heels and continue squeezing your shoulder blades. Repeat this sequence for a couple of breath cycles, then lower your arms and repeat the entire process three more times. Keep focusing on your breath and the alignment of your body as you embrace the openness and strength of this pose.

Goddess Pose Chair Side Stretch

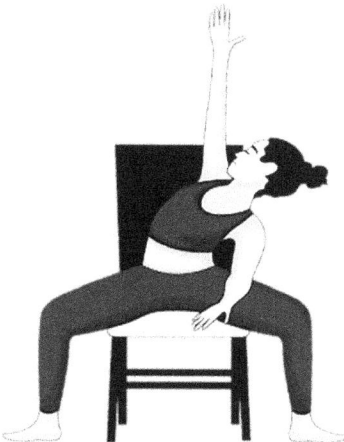

Open your legs wide with feet firmly grounded and pointing outward.

Place your right elbow on your right thigh, palm facing upward. Inhale and sweep your left arm up, gazing at your hand and looking up if possible.

Take three deep breaths in this position. Repeat the same sequence on the other side.

Chair Wide Legged Seated Twist

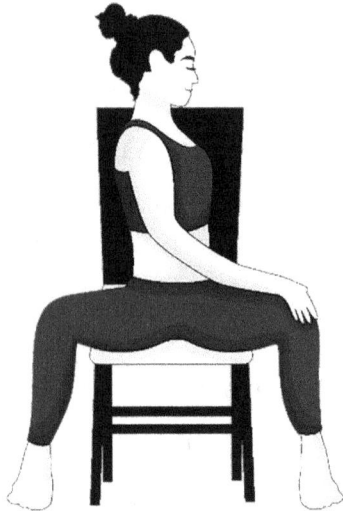

Remain seated in a goddess pose with arms lowered and with your knees wide open. Turn your toes slightly to face them forward and stack your knees over your ankles. Tuck your tailbone in. Both arms are resting on your thighs. Breathe in, lengthening your spine, and twist toward the right.

The twist begins in your belly, ribs, and chest. Your head is last to turn. The left hand goes onto your right knee and your right hand to the back of the chair. Breathe into the twist.

Stay here for three deep breaths. Exhale to release and return to the center. Repeat on the opposite side, each side twice.

Alternate Nostril Breathing Chair

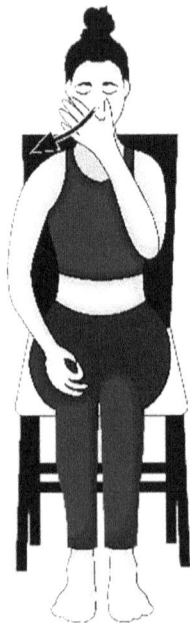

Sit nice and tall in a mountain pose. Rest your left hand on your left thigh or in your lap, or use it to support the elbow of your right arm. Close your right nostril with the thumb of that hand, inhale through the left, and then close it off with your ring finger and pinky. Exhale through the right nostril for a short pause before repeating this cycle three to five times with both nostrils. When finished, return to regular breathing.

When you finish this practice, sit with your eyes closed and your hands in your lap for a few minutes. Let your shoulders fall down and away from your ears. Check how you feel. Breathe in through your nose and exhale through your mouth. Breathe in and feel the air traveling through your throat and to your belly. Open your mouth and exhale.

Feel the sensations in your body right now. Warmth. Coolness. Tingling. Tightness. Pulsation. Relaxation. Hunger. Fullness. Observe the sensations in your body in this moment with patience and kindness. Explore both strong and subtle sensations with curiosity.

Day 6

SHOULDER, ARMS, AND WRIST EXERCISES

With today's well-rounded approach, you'll engage in targeted exercises that enhance the mobility and strength of your shoulders, arms, and wrists. You'll promote flexibility through gentle movements and stretches while building stability in these upper body areas. The routine includes poses to alleviate tension, improve range of motion, reduce muscle tightness, and enhance joint health.

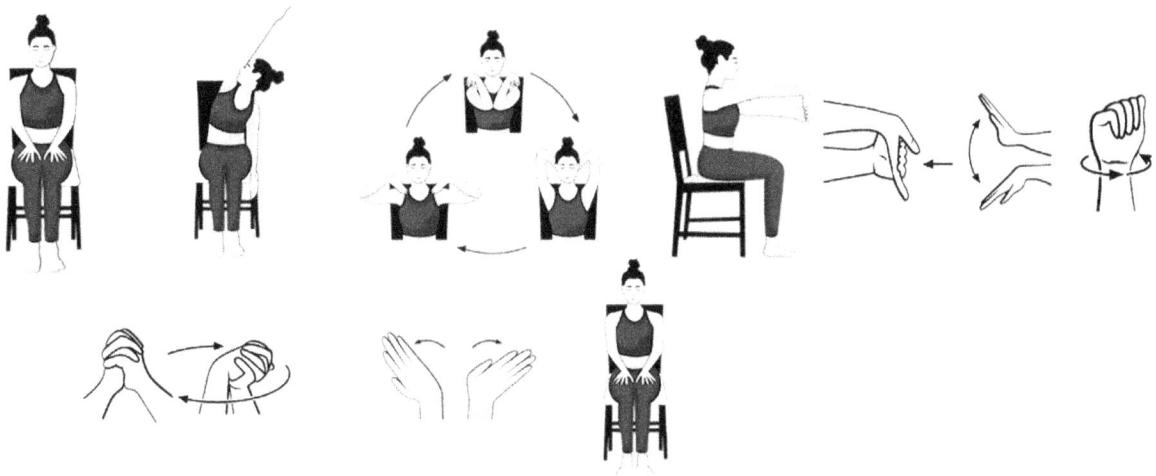

Begin in a mountain pose. You can lean to the back of the chair; however, keep your spine straight, shoulders lowered, and head above your heart. Keep your feet flat on the ground and your spine tall. Softly close your eyes or gaze downward to minimize distractions. Take a deep breath and exhale slowly. Start concentrating on your breath. Notice the sensation. Focus solely on your breath. Scan your body for any tension or discomfort, relaxing those areas with each breath. Engage your hands, moving them mindfully and feeling the sensations in your fingers and palms. Bring your focus back to your breath, following its natural flow in and out of your body. Visualize a warm, radiant light at a chosen point within your body, bringing tranquility to your entire being. Take a few more deep breaths, gradually returning your attention to the present moment. Open your eyes gently, taking a moment to appreciate the calmness and clarity you've cultivated.

Chair Seated Side Stretch Pose

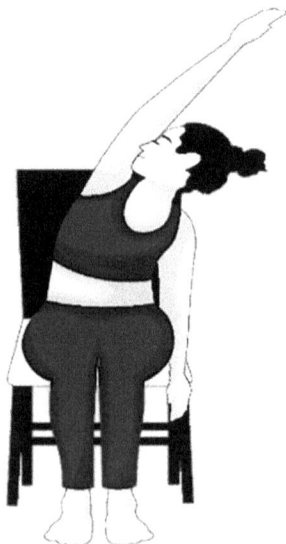

Sit upright. Place the hands on either side of the seat or your lap. Roll your shoulders down the back. Inhale and, pulling in the core, sweep the right arm above the head, creating a lateral bend on the left-hand side. Exhale into the stretch. Allow your chest and head to tilt to the left. Stay in this pose for three breaths.

On the inhale, return to the center. Repeat the same with the left side.

You can choose to stay on one side for two to three breaths before switching to the other side, or you may choose to move dynamically between one side and the other on the breath. Do what feels best for your body.

Shoulder Socket Rotation

Sit up tall with your back straight. Bring the fingertips to rest on the shoulders.

On the inhale, begin to move the bent elbows from the center, moving upward. Move them in a circular movement from the center about six times.

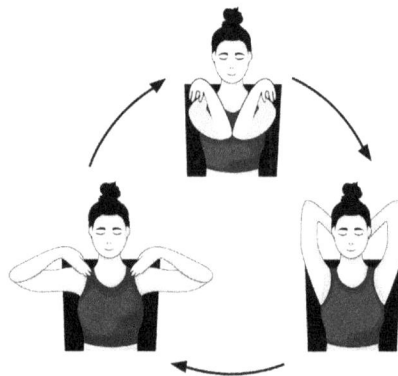

Repeat the opposite direction another six times. Watch your breath, and work on coordinating the action with your breath at your own pace. While practicing, pay attention to your breath and try to coordinate the movement with your breath at your own comfortable pace.

Wrist Flexion Stretch

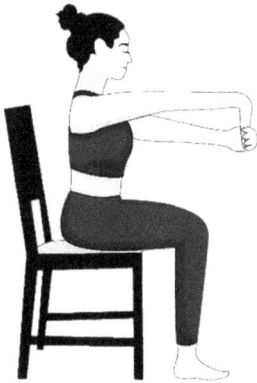

Inhale and extend your right arm straight out, palm facing down. Let your left hand take your right arm's fingers and gently pull them toward your chest. You may feel a stretch on top of your forearm. Stay here for three more breaths, gently going deeper into the stretch on each exhale while respecting your wrist's natural range of movement. Stretch as far as you comfortably can without pain.

Then, pull the fingers to the opposite side—fingers facing up. Repeat the same with your left arm.

Now inhale and extend your right arm straight out, palm facing and opened up. Let your left hand take your right arm's fingers and gently pull them toward your chest.

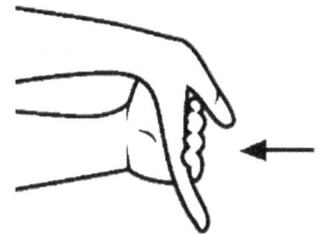

Carry on with wrist bending

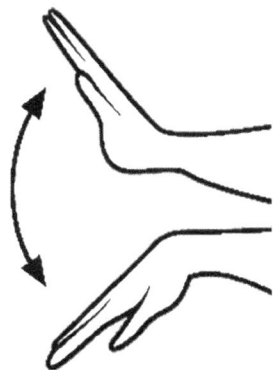

Bring the palms to face in the front with the fingers pointing upward.

Exhale, drop the fingers down as you flex the wrists of both hands. Inhale and raise them palm up, pointing the fingers up, and exhale to drop them down. Repeat this movement about six times, coordinating with the breath. Release and relax, bringing the arms down to the side, standing in mountain pose. Make sure the arms are stretched out and not bent at the elbows, and they are at shoulder level.

Wrist Joint Rotation

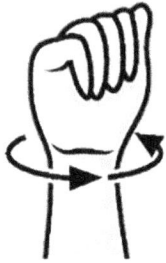

Rotate the right wrist clockwise—about ten times. Rotate the right wrist anticlockwise—about ten times. Repeat the same on the other side. Keep the arms stretched out.

Wrist Rolls Exercise Hands Clasped

Interlace your fingers and rotate your wrists gently at your own pace. Take a few low belly breaths here.

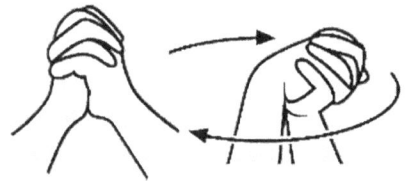

Wrist Exercise Side to Side Close Up

After rotating your wrists, point your fingers up straight, and move your wrist to the left and then to the right. Repeat for both hands. Breathe in and notice if your shoulders remain in the same position or try to move. Only the wrist should be

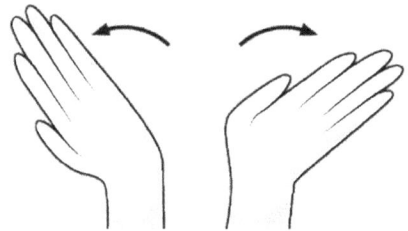

moving. Once the session is completed, close your eyes or soften your gaze. Notice your breath and how your body feels. Take a moment to thank yourself for carving out some time.

LOWER BACK, HAMSTRINGS, AND NECK RELAXATION

You'll target interconnected muscle groups of the lower back, shoulders, arms, hamstrings, and neck through gentle poses and stretches to release tension and promote a sense of ease. They often accumulate stress from daily activities.

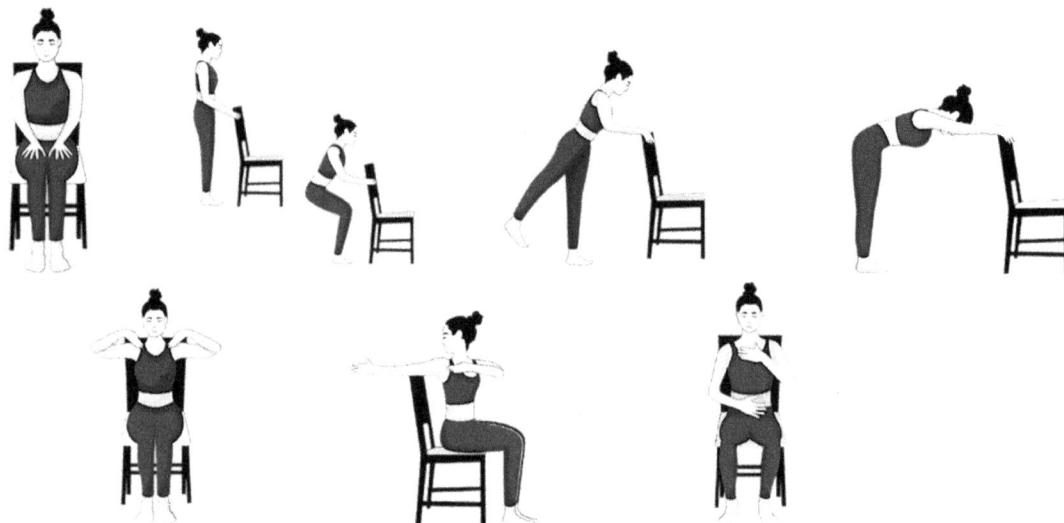

Mountain Pose Chair to Chair Pose Flow

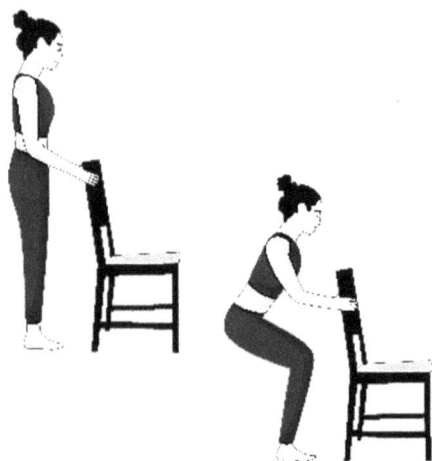

Stand at the back of the chair, holding onto the sides of the chair if help with balance is needed. Take a few deep breaths. Notice how you feel. Feel your ribs, inhale, and slowly exhale. Inhale, stand tall, grounding down into the soles of the feet and extending the spine upward. Exhale, sit weight back into heels. If you need a bigger challenge—your toes can be lifted to exaggerate the weight in the heels. Lower belly pulled in. The knees should be positioned behind the toes. Keep length in the spine and the back of the neck. Hold for three breaths. Repeat three times.

Mountain Pose Chair One Leg Backlit

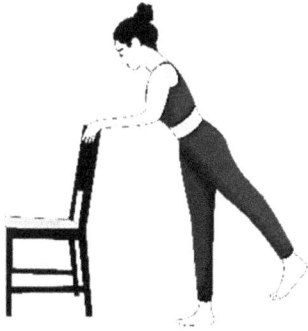

Keep your hands on the back of the chair. Stand tall. Bring your weight to the right foot. Extend the left leg back and lift off the ground. The toes of both feet are pointing forward. Move back and forth for three breaths, or you can hold it for three breaths. Repeat with the opposite leg. Repeat twice on each side.

Standing Forward Bend Chair

Stand in front of the chair in a standing mountain pose with your legs straight and fully stretched. Pull your kneecaps up. On the inhale, raise your arms toward the ceiling with your palms facing forward. Stretch your whole body. Take one or two breaths. On the exhale, bend forward from the waist. Keep your legs fully stretched.

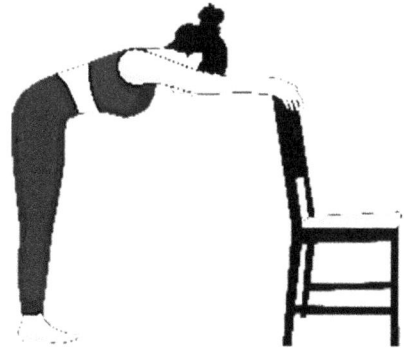

Make sure your body weight is placed equally on both feet. Keep the palms gently pressed, and do not push the body weight on the chair. Keep the length on the back, and fully extend the spine so that it is parallel to the floor. Hold the pose for three to five breaths. Repeat two sets of the practice.

Chair Seated Shoulder Circles

Sit on the chair facing forward, feet hip-distance apart or together on the floor. Inhale, lift your arms to the side, parallel to the floor. Exhale, and bring fingertips to shoulders. Begin to circle in one direction. Circles can be large or small. Pause, and bring attention to your breathing. Circle six to eight times in each direction. Keep your spine straight. Pause, inhale to open arms out, exhale lower arms down, and bring it to the center.

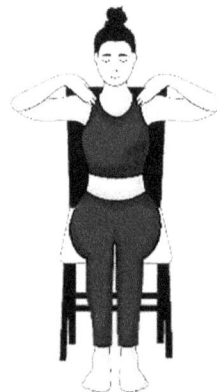

Seated Twist Arms Shoulder Level Pose Chair

Sit up nice and tall. Keep some distance between the chair's backrest and your back. Let the back be straight and long, feet grounded, and ankles and knees in one straight line. Keep the feet together or apart. Extend both arms to the sides in line with the shoulders, palms facing forward.

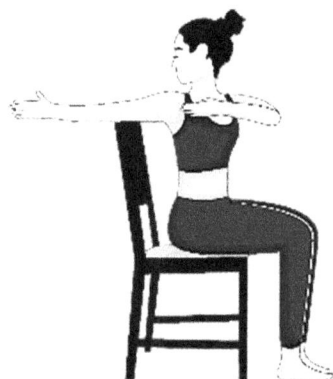

As you inhale, root the sit bones on the chair and lengthen the spine (imagine you are creating space between your vertebrae).

Exhale, twist to the right side originating from the lower back, taking the right hand to the back as far as possible and the left palm on the right shoulder.

Keep your gaze on the right hand by gently and comfortably turning the neck.

Stay here for three to five deep breaths. Keep twisting slightly more with every exhalation (as much as possible without any strain) without moving the lower body.

Mountain Pose

Find a comfortable seated position in the center of the chair, leaving some space between the back of the chair and your back. Rock back and forth until you locate your sit bones. Keep your feet hip-distance apart and flat on the floor. If you prefer, bring your knees together. Close your eyes or soften your gaze. Bring your attention to your breath, feeling the rise and fall of your chest and the expansion and contraction of your abdomen. Inhale deeply in and out. Inhale while counting to four, hold your breath for four, and exhale, counting to six. If these intervals are too long, do three, three, and four. Continue this rhythmic breathing for two minutes, allowing your body and mind to relax.

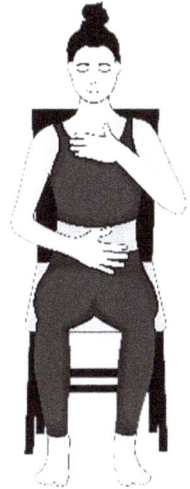

Day 8

HAMSTRINGS, HIP OPENERS, QUADRICEPS, AND UPPER BACK FLOW

Welcome to Day 8 of your chair yoga journey! This routine is designed to flow seamlessly through poses focusing on the hamstrings, heart openers, hip openers, quadriceps, and upper back. This sequence will nurture these vital muscle groups' flexibility, mobility, and balance.

The routine includes heart-opening poses to foster a sense of expansion and vitality, while hip and hamstring stretches promote ease of movement and reduce tightness. Quadriceps engagement and upper back stretch improve muscle functionality and posture.

You'll experience improved circulation, increased flexibility, and a deeper connection to your body through regular practice.

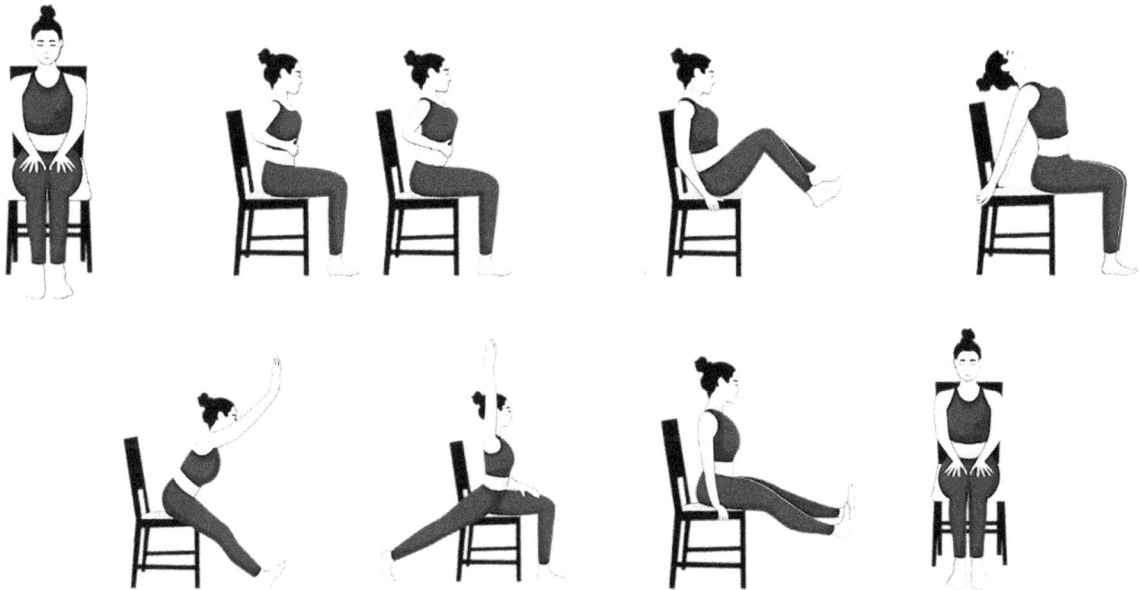

Seated Pelvic Tilt Tuck

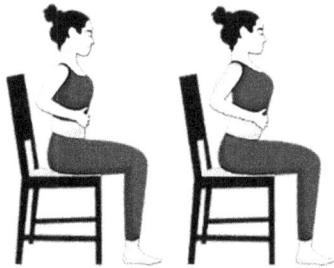

Place feet firmly on the floor in mountain pose, arms resting on your knees, and spine erect. Take a few deep breaths, put your arms on the tummy, and feel it rising and falling. Become aware of your surroundings. What can you hear? What can you smell? How do you feel? Are your shoulders lowered? Are your abdominals engaged? Do you feel the ground under your feet?

Place your hands on top of the pelvis crest to feel the movement. This is a slight movement, just tilting the tailbone back and forth. Inhale as you tilt the pelvis forward, like tipping a bowl full of water ahead. Exhale as you tilt the pelvis backward. Repeat for six to eight cycles.

Boat Pose Variation on Chair

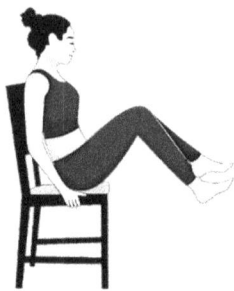

Sit straight and, on the inhale, grab the sides of the chair with your hands, positioning them right behind your buttocks. Curl your four fingers underneath the chair while resting your thumbs near the buttocks. Your weight should be on the outer edges of your palms. As you exhale, lift your feet off the floor while keeping your knees bent. Squeeze your inner thighs to keep your legs together and cross your ankles, aligning them with the chair seat.

Inhale and lengthen your spine as you engage your core and draw your abdomen to bear the weight of your legs. You'll naturally lean back, maintaining an open chest while using your hands on the chair for balance and reducing pressure on the lower back. Stay in this position for two to four breaths, rest, and repeat it again.

Cobra Pose Chair

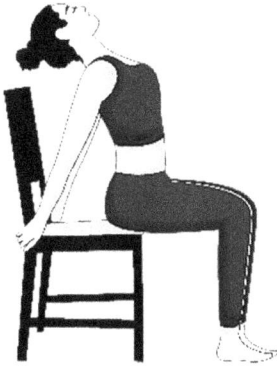

Begin by sitting up tall at the edge of the chair, ensuring your shoulders are relaxed. Open your chest and squeeze your shoulder blades together as you look upward.

Inhale deeply and take your arms behind you, holding onto the chair for support. Lift your chest and shoulders, gazing upward toward the sky with your chin slightly tilted. Remain here for three to six slow and deep breaths. If you like, repeat the sequence for a second round, staying in the pose for another set of breaths.

Seated Downward Facing Dog Pose Chair

Extend the legs—one at a time. On the inhale, flex the feet toward yourself. Extend the arms up, exhale to lean forward slightly from the hips, hugging the navel in. Think of keeping your back flat. Scoot the sit bones back to help balance. Keep the neck long. Bend your knees slightly if needed. Stay in this position for a few breaths. If required, take a break, and repeat it.

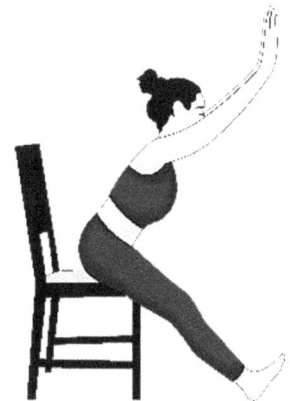

If this pose is not doable, with both legs stretched out, then alternate legs. Pay attention to the leg with more issues and try to hold that stretch a bit longer. After completing both legs, release the stretch and sit back, resting your feet on the floor.

Warrior Pose I Chair Variation

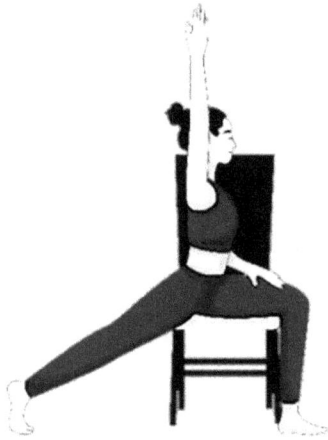

Slide your left leg toward the left side. Let the left leg rest over the edge of the chair while swinging your right leg behind you. Position the sole of your left foot on the floor, roughly parallel to the chair's seat. Straighten your right leg, using your toes for support. If needed, you can slightly bend your right knee. Your upper body is turned toward the left leg, creating a pleasing 90-degree angle with your knee stacked above the ankle. Engage your pelvis, ensuring a straight spine, and lift your heart upward. On an inhale, raise your right arm toward the ceiling while allowing your left forearm to rest on your thigh. Take two to three breaths and repeat on another side.

Staff Pose Chair

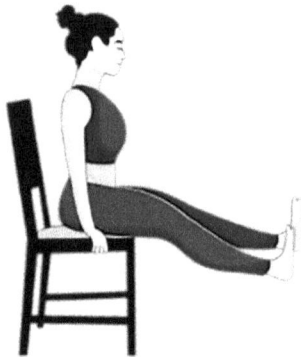

Sit upright with a straight spine and hold onto the sides of the chair seat with both hands. Engage your lower abdomen, and lift both legs simultaneously as you inhale. Keep your legs straight and parallel to the ground, flexing your feet upward. Wiggle your toes to keep your legs active, and if comfortable, hold this position for three breaths. If you cannot lift both legs simultaneously, try to alternate them. As you exhale, gently lower your legs back to the ground and return to a neutral seated position. Repeat it three times, resting in between.

Before you get on with your daily life, sit quietly and absorb the goodness of your practice.

EMPOWERING LOWER BACK, NECK, SHOULDERS, ARMS, AND UPPER BACK

Congratulations on reaching Day 9 of your chair yoga journey! Today's routine empowers and rejuvenates your lower back, neck, shoulders, arms, and upper back. With each movement, you're taking a step toward greater well-being and vitality.

As you engage in poses targeting the lower back, you'll strengthen and release tension, promoting a healthier spine. Gentle stretches for the neck, shoulders, arms, and upper back will melt away stress, fostering a sense of ease and relaxation.

Remember, every moment you dedicate to self-care is an investment in your physical and mental health. Embrace the challenge and embrace the rewards that this routine brings. As you move through the poses, visualize the energy flowing through your body, revitalizing each muscle group.

Stay committed, and you'll experience the benefits of increased flexibility, reduced discomfort, and improved posture. Your journey is a testament to your dedication to well-being, and each practice brings you closer to a more vibrant and balanced you. Keep up the great work!

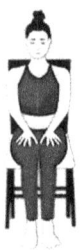

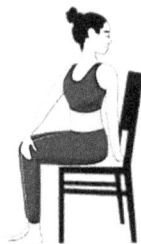

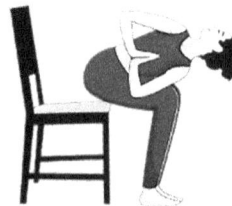

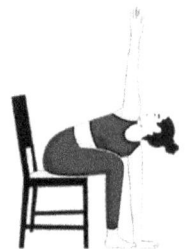

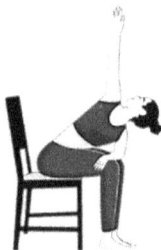

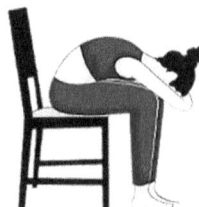

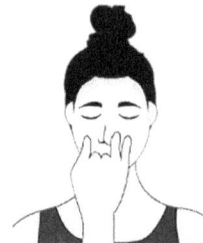

Sit nice and tall. Make sure you're not leaning on the back of the chair. Rock forward and back; find your sit bones. Sit tall with feet touching the floor and knees hip-width apart. Become aware of your breath, and when ready, move on to the next step.

Chair Seated Twists

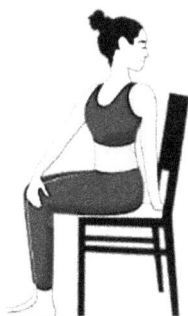

Inhale and place your arms over your head—lift and lengthen. With the exhalation, twist left from the base of the spine. Your ribcage, shoulders, neck, and eyes go to the left, but the hips remain on the chair. The right hand goes to the left knee, and the left hand is behind the left hip or on the back of the chair. Stay in the position for three deep breaths. Repeat the opposite side. Twice each side. Keep your shoulders away from the ears.

Revolved Chair Pose Hovering above Chair

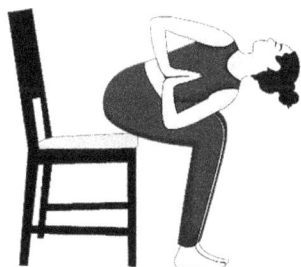

Breathe in as you stand firmly on your feet, gently bending your knees, with palms put together against your chest. Upon exhaling, gently lower your hips while maintaining a slight distance from the chair. Inhale again, and as you do, gracefully twist your chest and shoulders to the right, bringing your palms together in front of your heart.

Find yourself in the revolved chair pose, hovering over the chair for approximately three complete breath cycles. If you find it more comfortable, you can also perform this variation while seated on the chair. Once you've relished the sensation, smoothly transition to the other side, allowing the same sequence to flow in the opposite direction.

Revolved Chair Pose Chair

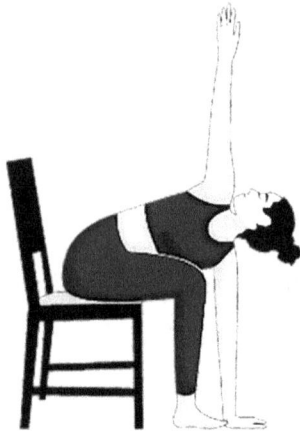

Start in a mountain pose with your spine straight and roll back the shoulders. Inhale and extend the spine, exhale, and bend forward, reaching for the ground with the left arm. Rest your palm on the floor; if this is not possible, lean onto your fingers or rest your left elbow on the top of your knees. The core is active and supports you, too. Inhale as you raise the right arm up and exhale, looking up at the extended limb. Stay here for two to three deep breaths and repeat on another side.

Seated Half Forward Fold Pose Chair

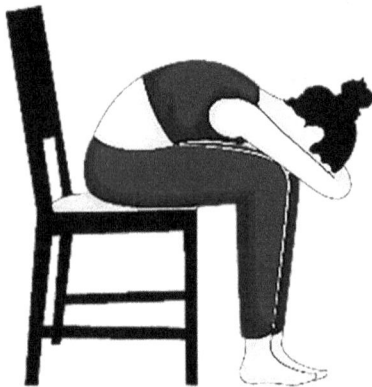

While seated in the mountain pose, breathe in deep for a few times to relax and extend the spine. Exhaling, fold your arms above your knees and allow your head to rest on your forearms. Feel your feet on the floor. Repeat this process as needed for a longer duration. If you need help, use a cushion for extra support under your chest and diaphragm. The aim is to release the tension and open the lower back. Breathe, listen to your body, and choose the position that you feel comfortable in. Stay for three to five breaths.

Alternate Nostril Breathing

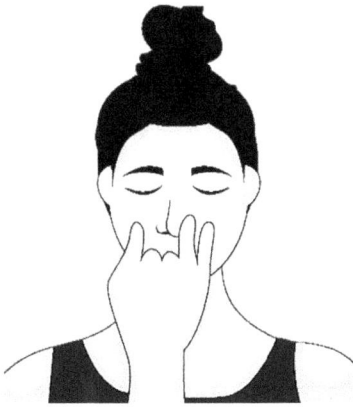

Sit comfortably in a mountain pose. Nadi shodhana, or alternate nostril breathing, is exactly as it sounds: breath control through breathing through alternating nostrils. The technique goes as follows:

Sit in a comfortable position. Each breath will be inhaled and exhaled through the nose. Bring your hand up to your nose, resting your thumb and ring finger on either side of your nose lightly without closing your nostrils. First, press your thumb against your right nostril, closing it. Exhale slowly and fully through your left nostril. Release your right nostril and press your ring finger against your left nostril, closing it. Inhale slowly and deeply. Release your left nostril and press your thumb back down on your right nostril. Repeat this process throughout the breathing exercise.

ABDOMINALS, HIP OPENERS, KNEES, QUADRICEPS, AND UPPER BACK REVITALIZATION

You've reached a milestone—Day 10 of your chair yoga exploration! Today's invigorating routine targets your abdominals, hip openers, knees, quadriceps, and upper back. This practice celebrates your commitment to self-care and your journey toward a healthier you.

Engage in poses that activate your abdominals, fostering core strength and stability. Explore hip openers that enhance flexibility and encourage a free flow of energy. Gentle stretches for knees, quadriceps, and the upper back create a harmonious blend of muscle care and revitalization.

You've come so far; this routine is a testament to your dedication. As you embrace these poses, embrace your journey—one that leads to increased vitality, reduced tension, and a deeper connection to your body. Keep moving forward with confidence and enthusiasm!

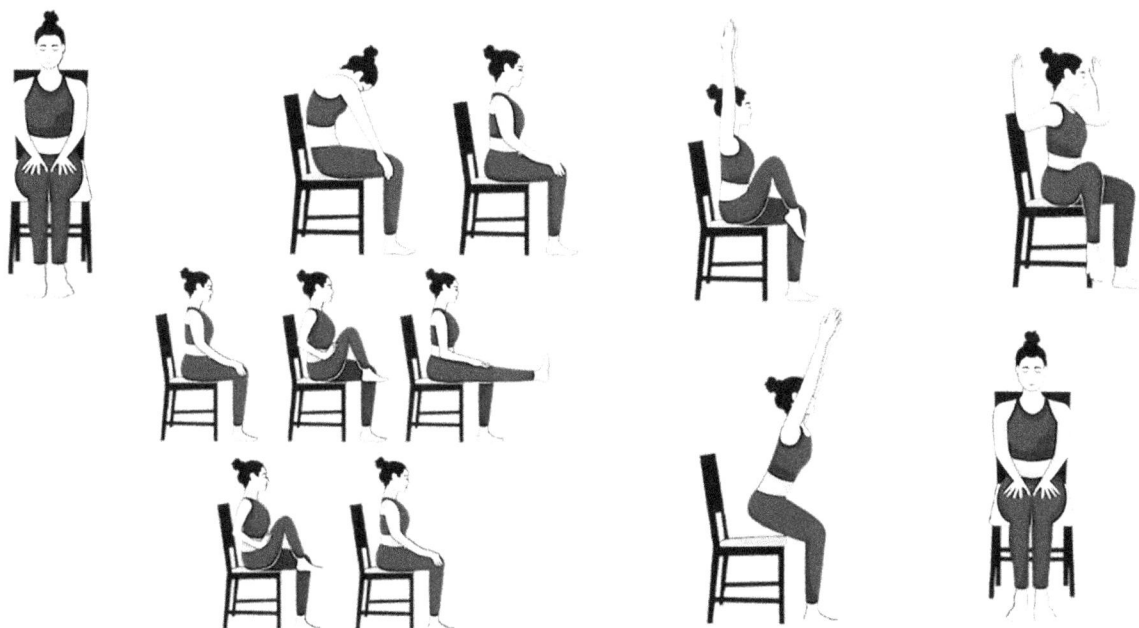

Before moving on to the cat-cow pose, let's practice left nostril breathing. We've already practiced right nostril breathing, so we will do the same—just with the left.

Left Nostril Breathing Variation Close Up: This breath practice of the left nostril enhances circulation to the right hemisphere of the brain, triggering heightened creativity, intuition, and emotional intelligence. Close the right nostril with the little finger and ring finger and breathe in and out through the left. Avoid if blood pressure is high. Do two rounds ten times each.

Chair Cat-Cow Pose

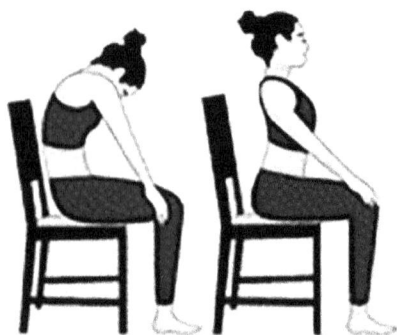

Place your arms on your knees.

As you inhale, expand your chest, allowing your head and chin to tilt slightly back. On the exhale, round your spine by curling your chest inward. Ensure your shoulders are relaxed, and be aware of the space between your shoulders and earlobes.

Practice coordinating your breath with the movement, moving at a comfortable pace. Repeat five to eight times.

Remember to smile, inhale deeply, and repeat this movement three to five times. Take your time and enjoy the practice.

Seated Low Lunge Variation Chair Arms Raised

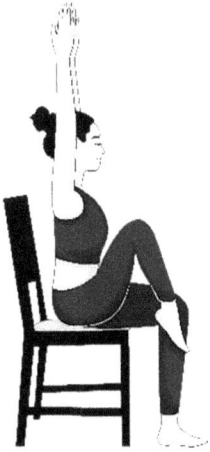

Sit tall with the spine extended. Engage your core. Notice all the muscles that take part in it when you cough. Engage the core with the belly button pulled in. Raise both your arms and lift one leg and exhale to lower the leg. Repeat the opposite side. Repeat six times for each leg.

Seated External Hip Rotation Pose Cactus Arms Chair

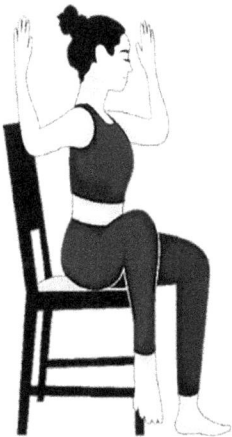

Sit upright, ensuring your shoulders are relaxed and your spine remains straight. Feel a sense of grounding through your hips and feet. Position your arms in a cactus shape, aligning your elbows with your shoulder and stacking your wrists above your elbows. Spread your fingers wide and direct them upward. Inhale, sweep your arms to the sides while keeping your elbows bent, as shown. As you breathe in, engage your core muscles, lengthen your neck, and draw your shoulder blades down your back.

With an inhale, extend your right leg to the right side, and as you exhale, bring it back to the center. Repeat this motion eight to ten times with one leg. If your arms feel fatigued, release the cactus arm position, and take a few breaths in the mountain pose. Then, repeat the sequence on the other side.

Seated Low Lunge Pose

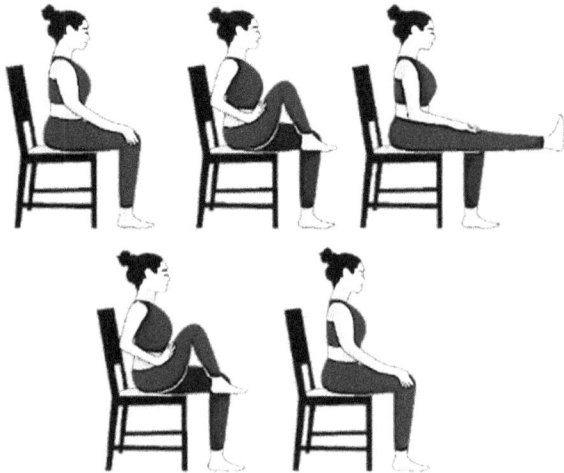

This easy flow will help stretch your feet, ankles, hips, and knees and strengthen your pelvic floor. Sit tall with both feet on the floor and sit bones grounded on the chair. Inhale, and bend your right knee toward your chest.

Exhale, and extend your leg out. Toes up toward the ceiling. Inhale, and bring it back by bending your right knee toward your chest. Exhale, and place your foot on the floor. Repeat on the other side—a total of five times for each leg. If you need to bend your knee toward your chest, you can grab under the knee and support your move.

Chair Pose Hovering Above Chair

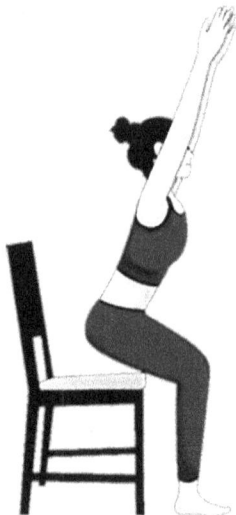

Maintain an upright posture and lift your arms above your head while exhaling deeply. Inhale and move into a chair pose, gently raising yourself to your feet above the chair. Inhale through your nose and exhale audibly through your mouth. Exhale and return to a seated position, arms still extended overhead. Inhale again and resume the chair pose. Repeat this sequence six times.

Come back to the chair mountain pose. Feel the ground under your feet.

Breathe in through your nose. Allow your lungs to fill with air. Feel your chest and abdomen rise as you inhale slowly and steadily. Hold your breath for a moment at the top of your inhale. Exhale through your mouth slowly. Focus on your sensations as you breathe—the rise and fall of your chest and the peaceful rhythm of your inhales and exhales. Let go of any thoughts or distractions, allowing your body and mind to relax. Absorb all the good of your session.

UPPER BACK, HIP, PELVIC, SHOULDER, AND ARM HARMONY

Welcome to Day 11 of your chair yoga series! This routine focuses on creating a harmonious balance in your upper back, hips, pelvic area, shoulders, and arms. You'll nurture these interconnected muscle groups through purposeful poses and stretches for improved well-being.

Experience gentle movements that address tension in the upper back, promoting relaxation and comfort. Hip and pelvic stretches encourage fluidity in movement and increased mobility. The routine includes shoulder and arm engagement, contributing to overall upper-body strength and alignment.

As you engage in this practice, please take a moment to connect with your body and its sensations. With each movement, you're promoting balance and vitality within yourself. Regular participation in these routines adds to your overall wellness journey, helping you create a more harmonious connection between body and mind.

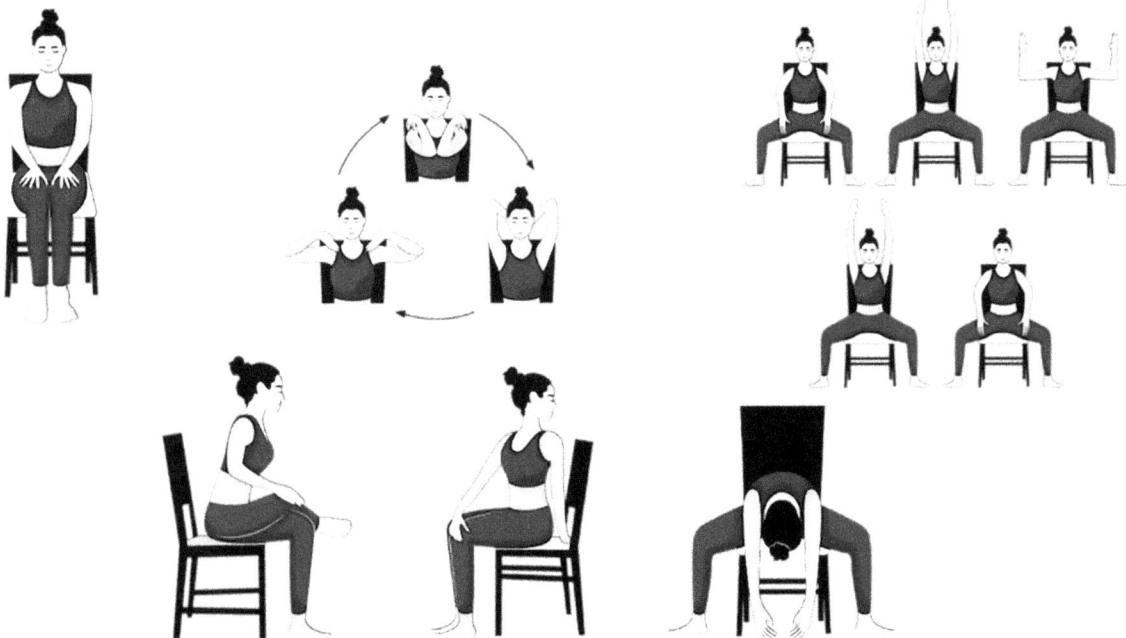

Mountain Pose

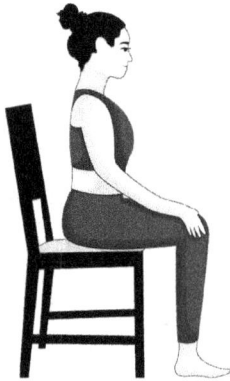

Find a comfortable seated position in the center of the chair, leaving some space between the back of the chair and your back. Rock back and forth until you locate your sit bones. Keep your feet hip-distance apart and flat on the floor. If you prefer, bring your knees together. Close your eyes or soften your gaze. Bring your attention to your breath, feeling the rise and fall of your chest and the expansion and contraction of your abdomen. Inhale deeply in and out. Inhale while counting to four, hold your breath for four, and exhale, counting to six. If these intervals are too long, do three, three, and four. Continue this rhythmic breathing for two minutes, allowing your body and mind to relax.

Shoulder Socket Rotation

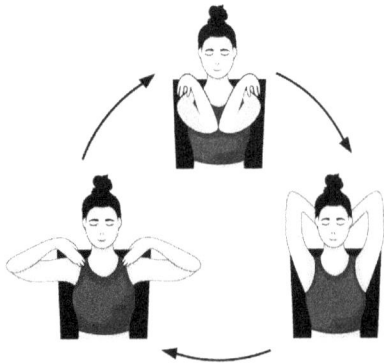

With the elbows bent, shoulder rolls strengthen the rotator cuff muscles, strengthening the shoulder joint. In addition to preventing injuries, this provides a solid foundation for poses requiring shoulder strength. Shoulder rolls with bent elbows can effectively aid in combating diseases and ailments caused by aging, such as osteoporosis and rheumatoid arthritis.

Move them in a circular movement from the center about six times. Repeat the opposite direction.

Goddess Pose on Chair Arms Flow

Inhale to rotate the hips outward, bringing the feet to 120 degrees, with toes pointing sideways and knees bent. Gently push out the inner thighs as you plant both feet firmly on the floor. Raise your arms overhead—palms facing each other—keeping shoulders away from ears. Exhale while bending elbows so forearms are perpendicular and palms are facing forward (cactus arms). Hold for three to fove breaths before inhaling to extend arms up again with palms together. Lower arms back down at shoulder level in an exhale, and place hands on inner thighs before inhaling again to raise them. Complete four to six repetitions of this flow, coordinating breathing as needed, then release and relax.

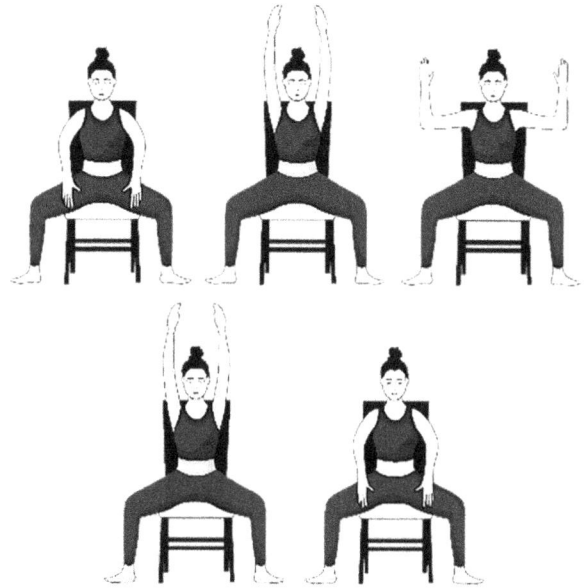

Chair Pigeon Pose

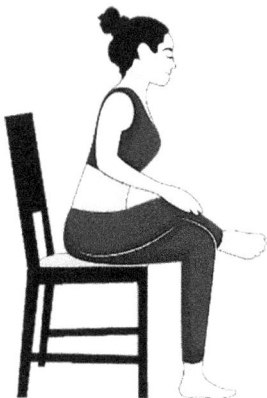

Sit nice and tall, with your back straight. Now, take a deep breath in as you lift your right leg, holding it gently with your hands, and position it over your left thigh, finding a comfortable sitting position. This seated chair pigeon pose serves to enhance the flexibility and fitness of your hip joint and knee through controlled movement. Once settled into the pose, aim to maintain an erect posture, and take three deep breaths or as many as you require to feel at ease. If you encounter difficulty in crossing one leg over the other, alternatively, lift your right leg, cradling it in your arms for a few seconds before gradually releasing it. Repeat this sequence on the opposite side. Repeat it twice on each side.

Chair Seated Twists

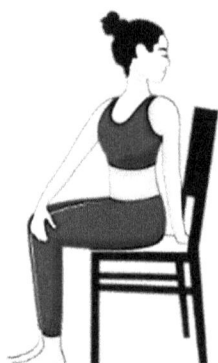

Make sure you're not leaning on the back of the chair. Rock forward and back; find your sit bones. Sit tall with feet touching the floor and knees hip-width apart.

Inhale and place your arms over your head—lift and lengthen. With the exhalation, twist left from the base of the spine. Your ribcage, shoulders, neck, and eyes go to the left, but the hips remain on the chair. The right hand goes to the left knee, and the left hand is behind the left hip or on the back of the chair. Stay in the position for three deep breaths. Repeat the opposite side. Twice each side.

Wide Legged Forward Bend Pose Chair Hands Floor

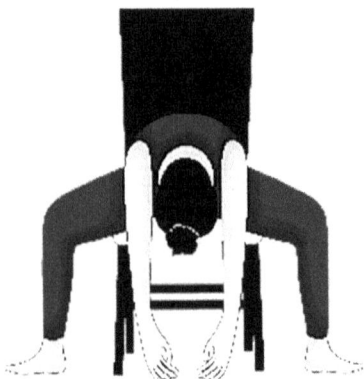

Open legs wide, keeping knees and toes in the same direction. Stack your knees over your ankles. Ground through all four corners of feet. Inhale and raise arms overhead. On the exhale, fold forward. Listen to your body and go as low as your body lets you. It doesn't matter if it's only a few inches. You can use blocks or a stack of books to bring the floor closer to you. Stay here for three deep breaths. If you're comfortable—remain for longer.

Let's complete the session with *Cooling Breath.*

Sit comfortably. Close your eyes gently if you're comfortable doing so, and take a few deep breaths to center yourself. Curl your tongue lengthwise into a "U" shape; if you can't, you can make an "O" shape with your lips. Inhale slowly and deeply through the curled tongue or lips as if you are sipping in cool air. Imagine that you are drawing in a refreshing breeze. After a full inhalation, close your mouth. Exhale slowly and thoroughly through your nose. Continue this cycle, inhaling through the curled tongue or lips and exhaling through the nose for 5 –10 breaths or as long as it feels comfortable. Feel the cooling sensation as you inhale and the calming effect as you exhale. After you've completed the *Cooling Breath* (Sitali Pranayama), return to normal breathing with your mouth closed.

PSOAS RELEASE FOR UPPER BACK COMFORT

On Day 12, you'll focus on nurturing your pelvic muscles and relieving your upper back. The psoas muscle is critical in connecting your upper and lower body, aiding in core stability, posture improvement, and overall movement.

This routine will help you to release tension in the shoulders and arms, promoting relaxation and flexibility. Addressing the psoas muscle benefits your upper back by alleviating stress on the spine, encouraging a balanced posture, and aiding in upper body movement coordination.

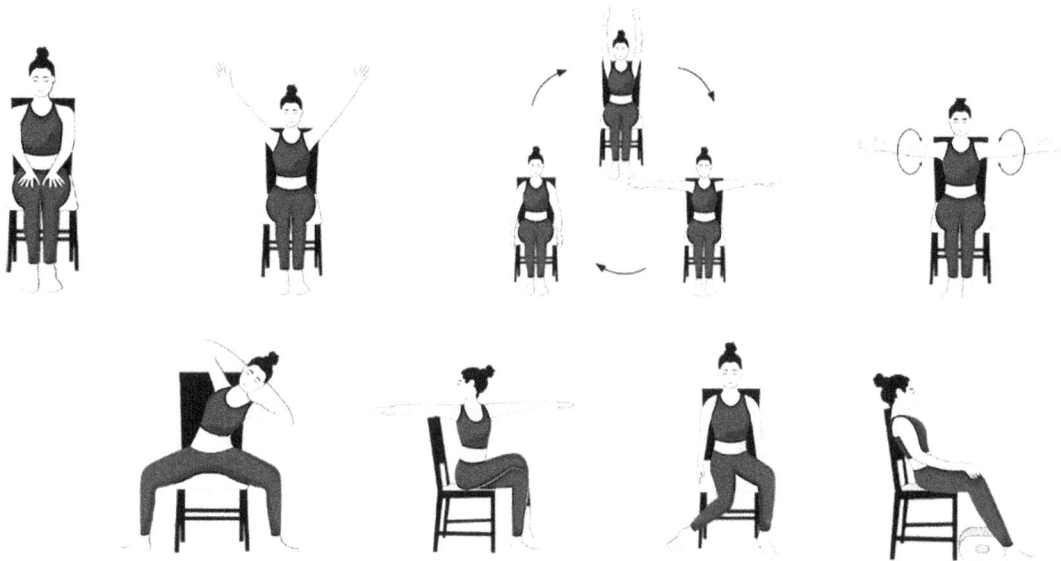

Seated Five-Pointed Star Pose Chair

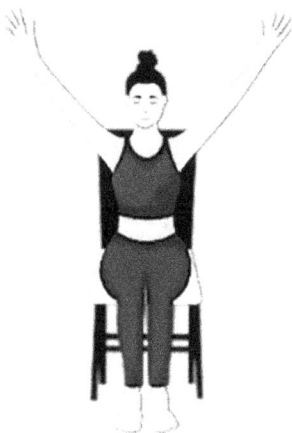

Take a seat in your chair and scoot forward, ensuring your feet rest flat on the floor. Straighten your back and elongate your spine. Tuck in your chin gently and draw your shoulders down while keeping your ears away from them. As you inhale, raise your arms up in a "Y" shape, spreading your fingers wide. As you exhale, slowly lower your arms and loosely clench your fists. Inhale again and lift your arms while spreading your fingers. Repeat this movement pattern five to seven times. Rest and repeat it again. Alternatively, you can lift your arms into a "Y" shape and hold that position for a few breaths before lowering them. Tune into your body and choose the option that brings comfort.

Chair Mountain Pose Sweeping Arms Flow

Sit in a mountain pose. Inhale, reaching the arms up, palms facing each other above your head. Exhale and slowly release them down, palms facing down. Inhale, reaching the arms up; exhale with palms facing down. Repeat the sequence for another five times.

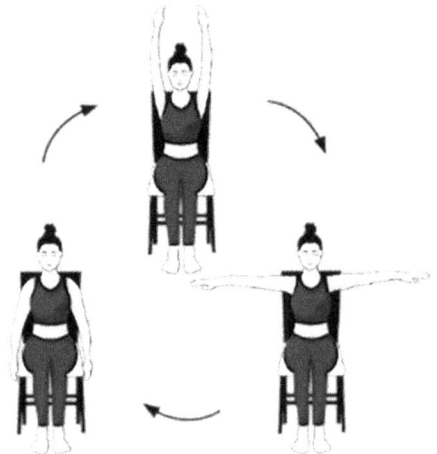

Arms to Side Rotations Chair

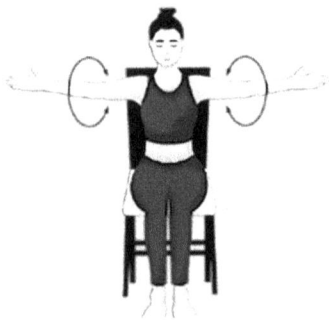

Raise your arms and spread them to the sides parallel to the floor, making a nice T. Breathe in and start making small circles with your wrists in one direction. After a couple of breaths, make a few circles in the opposite direction.

Start making small circles with your arms and slowly increase the motion, making them bigger, and then again, start rotating your arms in the opposite direction and making the circles small until you find stillness.

Goddess Pose Chair Hands behind Head Side Bend

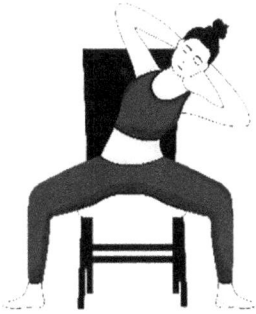

Lengthen your spine, relax your shoulders away from your ears, and settle into the goddess pose—knees and hips comfortably apart. As you breathe in, raise your arms overhead and position them behind your head. Extend away from the floor, maintaining open elbows. Inhale gently, drawing your shoulder blades slightly back. Upon exhaling, engage your core and bend to the right from your torso. You can pause in this position for one or two breaths, or return to the center with your inhale before repeating. Exhale and switch sides. Carry out several rounds on each side for a complete experience.

Seated Revolved Arms Extended Eagle Legs Pose

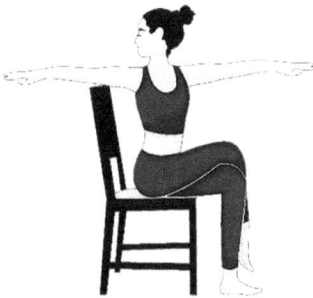

Sit up nice and tall. Pull the shoulders away from the ears and roll the shoulder blades back. Put your right leg over your left leg. On the inhale, lift your heart to the sky. Extend your arms to a T, and on the exhale, twist your torso to the right, the head looking over your right shoulder, arms being straight, at the shoulder level, parallel to the floor. Stay in the pose for three breaths. On the exhale, release. Repeat on the other side.

Seated Windshield Wiper Pose Chair

This movement will help you to loosen up your hips and knees. Sit up straight and tall. Keep your legs wide apart. Take a few breaths to the windshield wiper, your knees in and out, moving side to side with your breath at your own pace, releasing the tension. Come back to the center.

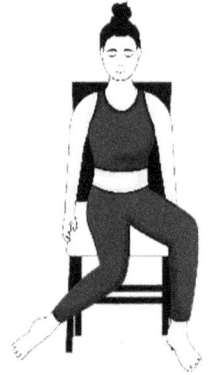

Seated Corpse Pose Chair Legs Bolster

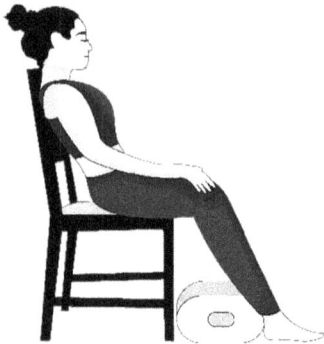

As you conclude your practice, take a moment to sit with your eyes gently closed and your hands resting in your lap. If you need one, use a bolster or make one yourself by rolling up a big towel or a cover. Allow your shoulders to naturally relax, easing away from your ears. During this transition into the rest of your day, take the time to absorb all the beautiful benefits of the poses you've just experienced.

Check in with yourself and notice how you feel. Take a deep breath in through your nose, feeling the air travel down your throat and into your belly. Exhale gently through your mouth. Continue this mindful breathing for a couple of minutes, allowing yourself to fully connect with the present moment.

Before you begin moving into the activities of your day, take a few more minutes to absorb the goodness of your practice. Observe your body with a sense of curiosity and acceptance, free from any judgment or effort to change anything. Be fully present, noticing the sensations that exist in this moment.

ABDOMINALS, FEET AND ANKLES, HIPS, AND LOWER BACK WELLNESS

Welcome to Day 13! Engage in abdominal exercises to strengthen your core, which aids in improving posture and supporting better spinal alignment. Addressing feet and ankles promotes better mobility, supporting overall body movement for effective workouts. Hip stretches create flexibility, which is essential for a balanced exercise routine. Lower back activities alleviate tension and discomfort, ensuring you're ready for active sessions.

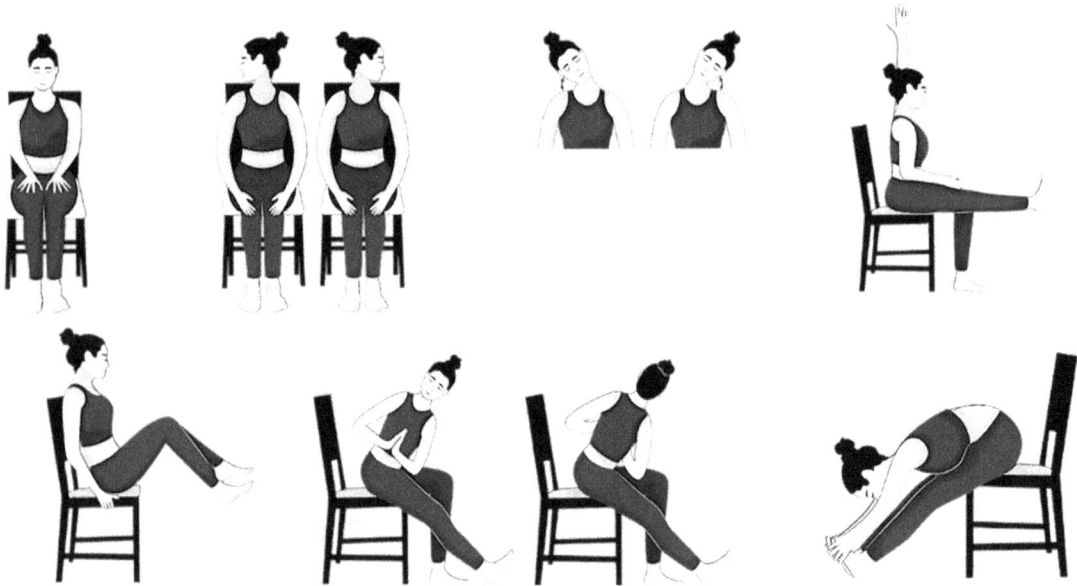

Chair Neck Rolls

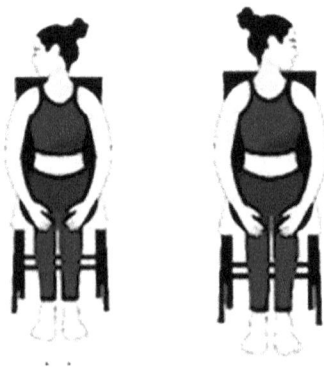

Sit up in a mountain pose to begin your session. Find your center, and take a few relaxed breaths. Inhale, elongate your spine, and feel your sit bones grounding while envisioning the crown of your head reaching upward. Tuck your chin slightly. Inhale, and turn your head to the right, then exhale. Inhale back to center, exhale, and pause before switching sides. Repeat on the other side. Complete this sequence two to four times on each side.

Don't try to lift your shoulder to the ear. You bend your neck as far as your body allows today. Sit tall and straight with your head stacked over your heart and your heart over your hips. Feel your feet firmly placed on the ground, hip-distance apart. Leave some space between you and the chair's back.

Inhale, move your ear toward the left shoulder, relax, and exhale. Then, inhale and return to the center. Repeat this movement from neck/ear to shoulders while coordinating breath and movement. Repeat the movement three to five times on each side.

Easy Pose Chair One Leg Opposite Arm Raised

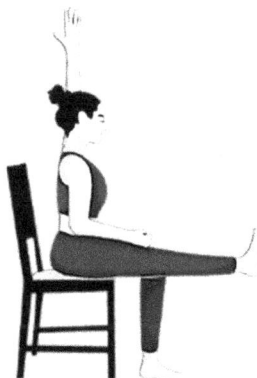

Sit nice and tall, away from the chair back. Use your ocean breath if you can.

Engage your core, and pull the belly button in toward the spine. Inhale and raise the right leg and left arm. Hold for a few breaths. Feel how your leg is activated. Lower the leg, or bend through the knee if it's too challenging. Remember to breathe and coordinate movement with breath. Release to the ground after a couple of breaths. Repeat two to three times for each side.

Boat Pose Variation on Chair

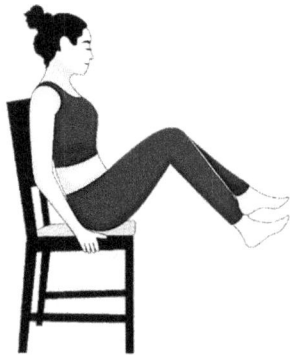

Sit straight and, on the inhale, grab the sides of the chair with your hands, positioning them right behind your buttocks. Curl your four fingers underneath the chair while resting your thumbs near the buttocks. Your weight should be on the outer edges of your palms. As you exhale, lift your feet off the floor while keeping your knees bent. Squeeze your inner thighs to keep your legs together and cross your ankles, aligning them with the chair seat. Inhale and lengthen your spine as you engage your core, and draw your abdomen to bear the weight of your legs. You'll naturally lean back, maintaining an open chest while using your hands on the chair for balance and reducing pressure on the lower back. Stay in this position for two to four breaths, rest, and repeat it again.

Sage Twist I Pose Chair Prayer Hands

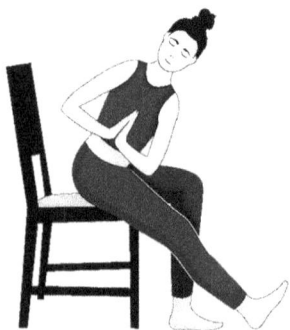

Scoot to the front edge of your chair. Join your palms together at your chest's center in a prayer position. Bend your left leg at a 90-degree angle while extending your right leg, pulling the toes toward you. Maintain a straight spine and an elongated neck. As you exhale, slowly rotate your upper body to the right, inclining forward. Experience the stretch in your calves and back. Hold this pose for three to four breaths. Exhale, and return your upper body to the center.Repeat the same on the opposite side. Repeat twice on each side.

Supported Seated Forward Bend Pose Chair against Wall

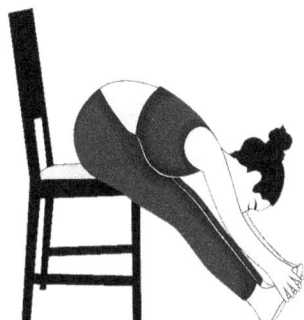

Bring the back of your chair to a wall for support so that the chair doesn't move. Sit toward the edge of the chair. Extend the legs out in front of you. On the inhale, raise your arms, and on the exhale, fold forward till you feel a stretch. There is no need to force your body to go deeper. Hold the position for five full breaths or less. Gently return to a neutral position.

Before completing the routine and continuing with your daily activities, remain seated in a mountain chair position and absorb the practice.

Take a few deep, cleansing breaths. Inhale slowly through your mouth and exhale through your nose. Notice how you feel. Observe your breath. Let each breath flow effortlessly, like the gentle rise and fall of the tide. As you breathe, visualize a sense of calm and tranquility wash over you like a soothing wave. Imagine this peace enveloping your entire being, from the top of your head to the tips of your toes.

Stay in this state of mindfulness for a few moments, savoring the stillness and serenity you've cultivated through your chair yoga practice. When you're ready, gently open your eyes, carry this inner calm, and continue your day with renewed energy and relaxation.

HIP OPENERS, LOWER BACK, AND NECK RELIEF WITH CORE ACTIVATION

Today's sequence focuses on hip openers, lower back comfort, and neck relief. Additionally, I introduced the eagle arms pose, which enhances upper body flexibility and activates your core muscles, contributing to overall strength and stability. With each movement, envision tension melting away and muscles awakening.

You'll find increased mobility, reduced discomfort, and a stronger core through consistent practice. Your commitment to self-care is evident in your dedication to these routines. Keep showing up.

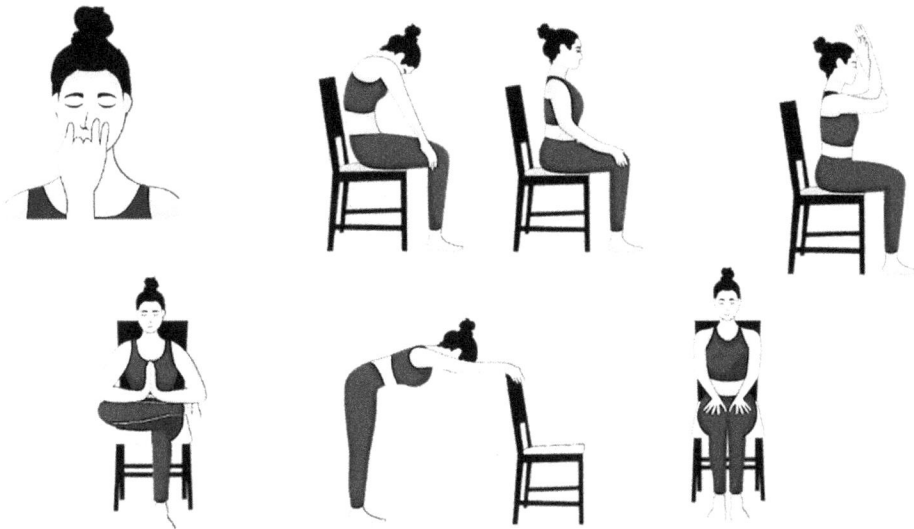

Alternate Nostril Breathing Chair

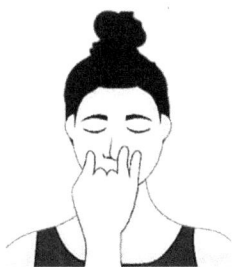

Sit nice and tall in a mountain pose. Rest your left hand on your left thigh or in your lap, or use it to support the elbow of your right arm. Close your right nostril with the thumb of that hand, inhale through the left, and then close it off with your ring finger and pinky. Exhale through the right nostril for a short pause before repeating this cycle three to five times with both nostrils. When finished, return to regular breathing.

Chair Cat-Cow Pose

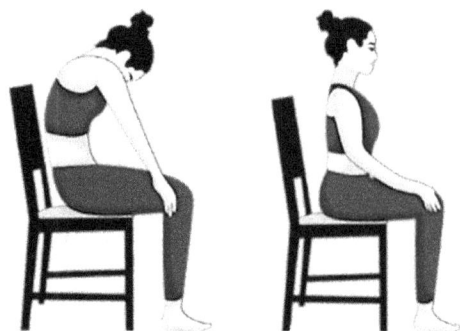

Place your arms on your knees. As you inhale, expand your chest, allowing your head and chin to tilt slightly back. On the exhale, round your spine by curling your chest inward. Ensure your shoulders are relaxed, and be aware of the space between your shoulders and earlobes. Practice coordinating your breath with the movement, moving at a comfortable pace. Repeat five to eight times.

Remember to smile, inhale deeply, and repeat this movement three to five times. Take your time and enjoy the practice.

Eagle Arms

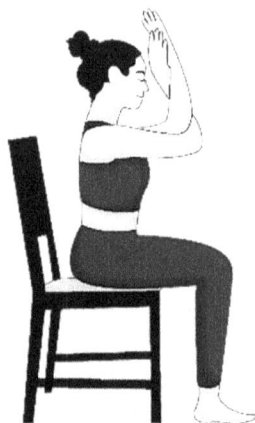

This movement offers a swift means of alleviating shoulder and neck stiffness by stretching the entire back muscles. Find a comfortable seat on a chair, ensuring your back is straight and your feet are securely planted on the floor. Take a few calming breaths in this position. Cross your elbows, placing your right arm over the left.

Link your arms together, and focus on your breath as you hold the position for three breaths. Release and replicate the movement on the other side. Cross your left elbow over the right. Maintain your breath for another three breaths. Then, release and return to the center. Repeat it twice.

Chair Pigeon Pose Variation Forward Bend

On the inhale, bring the right ankle to rest on the left thigh with your hands, keeping the knee in line with your ankle as much as possible. The left leg is grounded with the flat foot in the chair pigeon pose. Use both hands to adjust the ankle position on the other knee. Breathe and lengthen the spine. Feel the hip flexors contracting and the joints of the hips, knee, and ankle being active. Engage the pelvic floor muscles and remain here for about four to five breaths, consciously pushing the right knee down (but without using the hands). Inhale, and bring the hands in front of your chest, palms facing each other. Keep forearms parallel to the ground. As you exhale, go for a forward bend from the hips to intensify the stretch. Engage the pelvic muscles. Try bringing the chest closer to the thighs. Breathe, and observe how your body feels—moving forward when exhaling. Find the spot until you can't go any farther, and once comfortable, hold for about three to four breaths. If you can, on the exhale, go deeper into the forward bend. If you cannot, then stay where you are. Remember to keep your spine long, your shoulders relaxed, and away from your ears. To release, inhale, lift your head, and come up to straight back, exhale, release the hands, and with the support of hands, release the right leg, and relax. Repeat the same steps on the other side.

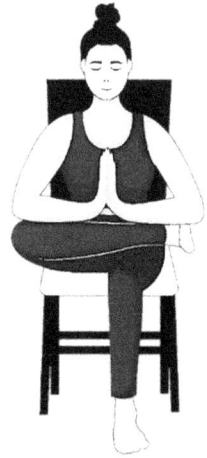

Standing Forward Bend Chair

Begin in the mountain pose, elongating your legs and engaging your kneecaps. Extend your arms toward the ceiling with palms facing forward, creating length throughout your entire body. Fold forward from the hips with an exhale, ensuring your legs are extended without locking the knees. Place your palms lightly on a chair about three feet before you. Maintain a parallel alignment between your spine and the floor while gently lifting through your sitting bones. Remember, the chair offers support, but avoid putting all your weight on it. Feel your abdominal muscles engaging to maintain your posture and spinal alignment. Sense the energy radiating through the back of your legs and ensure even pressure on both the inner and outer edges of each foot. Hold this pose for thirty to sixty seconds, gradually aiming for longer durations as you progress. Throughout the practice, maintain steady and even breathing.

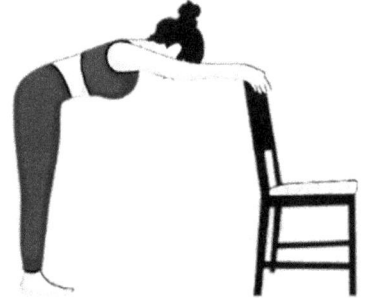

HAMSTRINGS, HIPS, KNEES, AND QUADRICEPS CARE

Today, you will work on your hamstrings, hips, knees, and quadriceps. You'll promote flexibility and strength in these interconnected muscle groups through a sequence of purposeful poses.

Engage in gentle movements that address tightness in the hamstrings, promoting better leg flexibility. Hip- and knee-focused exercises encourage mobility and joint health, while quadriceps stretches enhance overall leg functionality.

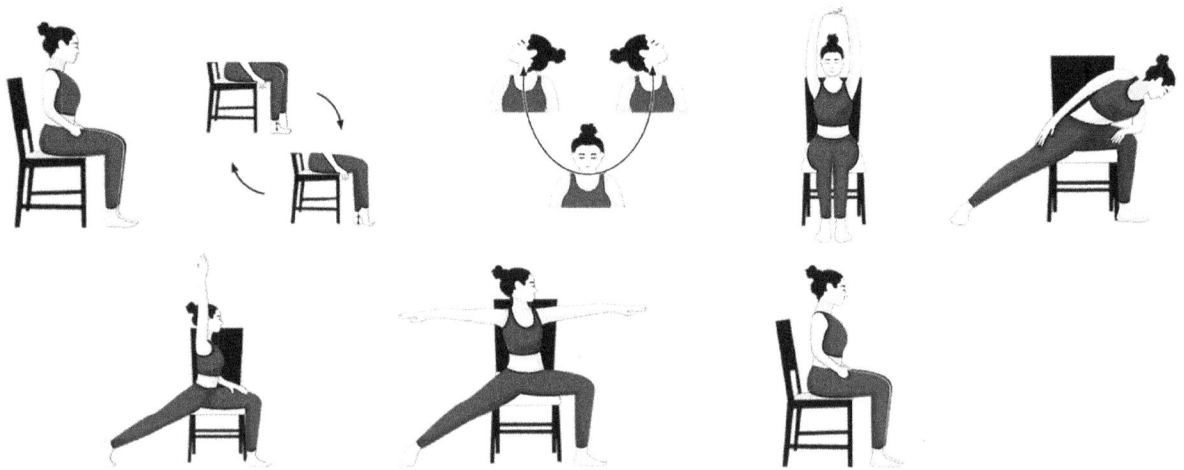

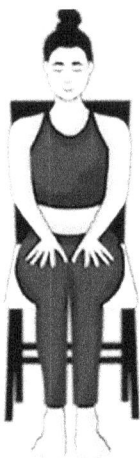

Sit comfortably on the chair and maintain a straight spine. You can lean on your chair backrest—as long as you sit tall with your shoulders lowered. Unbend your arms and stretch out your fingers. This is to imitate a lion's claws. Inhale through the nostrils, then exhale with a loud "ha" from the mouth, extending your tongue as close to the chin as you can. While breathing out, focus on the middle of your forehead or the end of your nose. Fill up with breath, and go back to neutral facial expression. Repeat four to six times.

Chair Mountain Pose Heel Raise

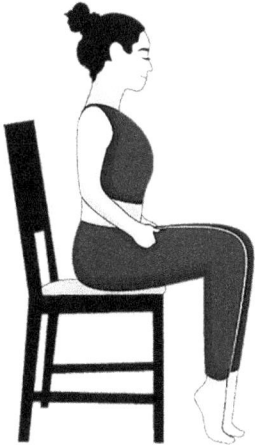

Start with feet flat on the floor. Inhale—lift both heels, pressing the toes into the floor, and lower on the exhale. Repeat five times. Inhale—lift the right heel, pressing the toes into the floor, and lower on the exhale. Repeat five times.Continue by lifting your toes. Inhale—lift your right toes, pressing your heels into the floor and lower on the exhale. Repeat the same with your left foot. Repeat five times for each foot. Lift the toes of both feet at the same time, pressing the heels into the ground. Repeat another five times. Use your deep breath.

Neck U Rotation Close-Up

While the movement may seem simple, the improved range of motion helps with other poses and day-to-day activities. Sit comfortably in the chair with a straight spine and feet on the floor. Let your arms rest at your sides. As you inhale, turn your head to the left, exhale, and tuck your chin toward your chest. Inhaling once more, move your chin toward the right shoulder, and exhale, rolling it back to your chest. Alternate between both sides until you return to a neutral position with the chin parallel to the floor. Stay here for two rounds.

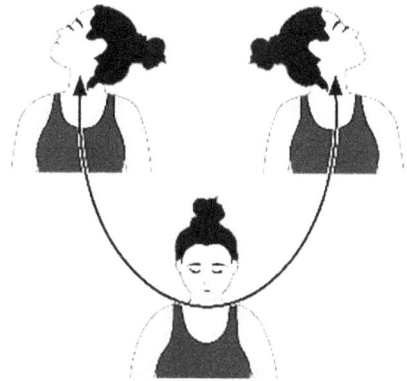

Chair Upward Hand Stretch Pose

On the inhale, raise your arms above your head and bring the hands in an interlock. On the exhale, try to lower your shoulders. Think about making the spaces between your ears and shoulders. Remain in a stretch position for two to three breaths. Release your arms on the exhale.Repeat it twice.

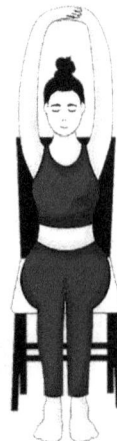

Extended Side Angle Pose Variation Elbow Chair

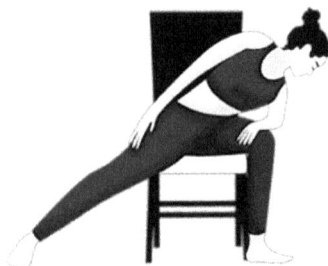

On the inhale, sit sideways, resting the left thigh on the chair while bringing the other leg out. Exhale, stretch the right leg out, and place the right foot on the floor with toes facing forward. Inhale—adjust the left foot, turning it outward, and rest the left hand on the left thigh. Let your right arm rest on the right thigh. Exhale, rotate your chest, and face downward, gazing toward the left side of the ground. Don't let your torso collapse; keep it straight. Stay for three to four breaths. Repeat on the opposite side.

Warrior Pose I Chair Variation

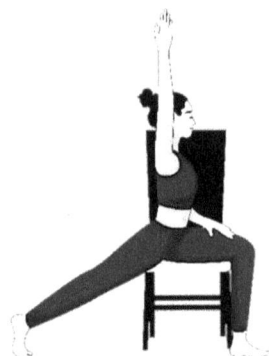

Slide your left leg toward the left side. Let the left leg rest over the edge of the chair while swinging your right leg behind you. Position the sole of your left foot on the floor, roughly parallel to the chair's seat. Straighten your right leg, using your toes for support. If needed, you can slightly bend your right knee. Your upper body is turned toward the left leg, creating a pleasing 90-degree angle with your knee stacked above the ankle. Engage your pelvis, ensuring a straight spine, and lift your heart upward. On an inhale, raise your right arm toward the ceiling while allowing your left forearm to rest on your thigh. Stay for three to four breaths. Repeat on the opposite side.

Warrior Pose II Chair

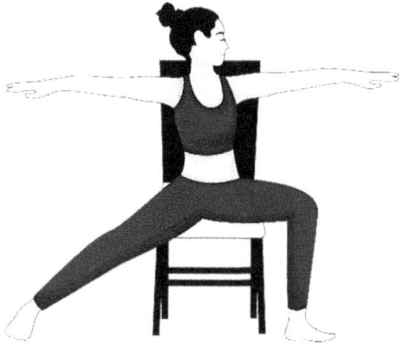

Sit on the edge of the chair. Inhale, and separate the feet. Starting on the left first, open the left leg like a goddess pose, but the left leg only. The knee aligns with the ankle and hip, forming a 90-degree angle. The foot is flat and relaxed, with the toes pointing to the left. Exhale and extend the right leg behind to make it straight in the knee. The right foot is flat here, and the toes point to the front. Make your back straight with your hands resting on the knees. Sit nice and tall. Once the body is comfortable, inhale and extend your arms at shoulder level to a nice T. Ensure the palms are face down and elbows are not bent. Finally, turn your head and gaze at your left fingers. Don't collapse; the torso is straight, and the shoulders are lowered. While here, check the alignment of the legs—the front knee doesn't drop to the side. Stay balanced in the pose. Breathe slowly, deeply, and softly. Stay for three to four breaths.

To release the pose: Turn your head back to the center on the exhale. Lower your hands, and realign your legs to the mountain pose. Stay here for a while. Following the previous steps, counter the stretch on the other side.

To cool down, finish your practice in a mountain pose. Feel the rise and fall of your abdomen with each inhale and exhale. Do five rounds, and feel the ground under your feet. Move your toes and feel each of them. Notice how you feel. Move your fingers and wrist. Observe. Observe your breath. Concentrate on it for a few minutes and, when you're ready, then finish the session.

FEET AND ANKLES RENEWAL — COMPLETING A BALANCED JOURNEY

Welcome to Day 16 of your chair yoga series! Today's routine focuses on renewing your feet and ankles, adding the final touch to a well-balanced journey covering various body parts.

As you engage in gentle stretches and movements for your feet and ankles, you're providing much-needed care to these foundational components of your body. Remember that your feet and ankles support you daily; this practice is your way of expressing gratitude to them.

By addressing these often-neglected areas, you're completing a comprehensive journey that has targeted different muscle groups. Throughout these routines, you've nurtured flexibility, strength, and relaxation in various parts of your body.

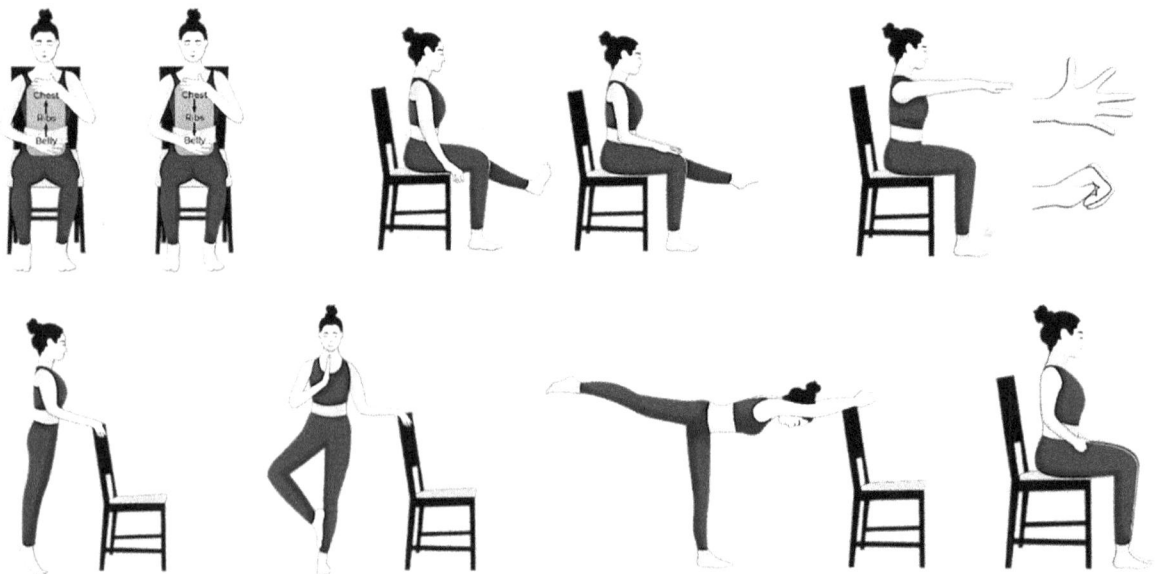

Start in a mountain pose. Feel the rise and fall of your abdomen with each inhale and exhale. Do five rounds, and feel the ground under your feet. Move your toes and feel each of them.

Three Part Breathing

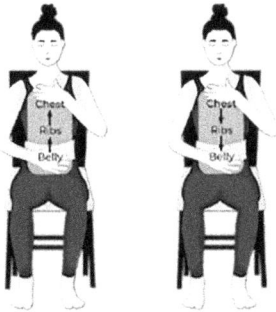

To end the routine, let's practice a breathing exercise. As you begin, you may place your hands on different body parts to feel the air expanding and contracting the area. Begin by inhaling air into your belly, allowing it to expand with each breath in and flatten with each exhale. Take your time to get comfortable with this motion.

Next, take a deep belly breath, and when your belly is expanded, draw in another small breath and focus it into your lower chest. Place your hand on your lower chest to feel it expand. When exhaling, first release the air from your chest, then from your belly, allowing both to deflate completely. Practice this until you feel comfortable with the movement.

Now, breathe into your belly, then into your lower chest, and finally, draw in one last breath to fill the upper chest, expanding it up to the collarbone. Feel your entire chest fully expand. When exhaling, start by releasing the air from your upper chest, then from your lower chest, and finally from your belly. Let each part deflate completely before moving on to the next.

Chair Flexing Foot Pose

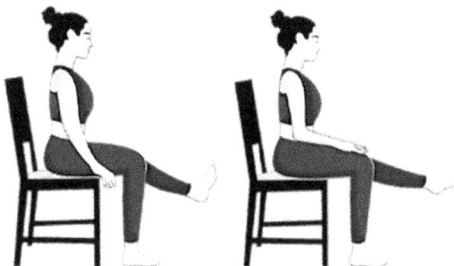

Draw the crown of your head towards the sky and lengthen your spine. Place your hands gently on your knees. Begin by lifting the right leg and pointing the toes away from you. Inhale, lift your toes towards your face, and press the heel away. Exhale and point out the toes. Repeat a couple of rounds before switching the legs. Repeat on the left side. Repeat each leg four to six times. This is a great movement to increase blood flow to the lower extremities of the body, which can aid in reducing leg lymphedema, varicose veins, and other possible discomforts in the calves and feet.

Hand Clenches Chair

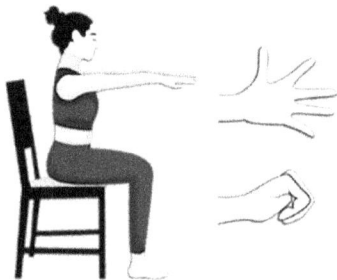

Stretch the arms out and sit up nice and tall. Lift straight arm within shoulder level. Stretch all the fingers out wide open. Close them to make a fist. Breathe deeply. Keep stretching your fingers out and returning them to a fist fifteen times. Take a rest and repeat it.

Heel Raises Chair

Use the chair's support when attempting heel raises if balance poses a challenge. As you inhale, elevate your body, finding equilibrium on your toes, experiencing the sole's gentle stretch. This sensation extends from the hips, emphasizing a seamless connection to the leg stretch as you gradually rise. Maintain this posture for three to six breaths, then release and repeat. If this is too challenging, you can go up and down, as this is also a great way to stretch your feet.

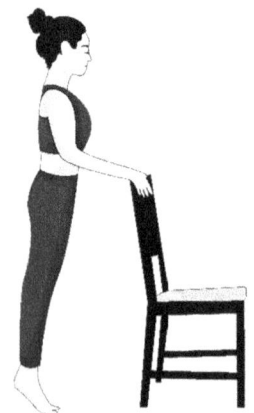

Beginner Tree Pose Chair

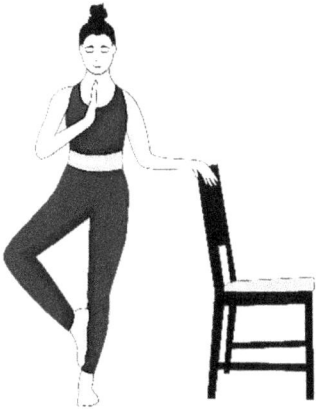

Standing with one hand on the chair for balance, start shifting weight onto the right leg. Ensure your hips stay still. Find a point to gaze at in front of you. Slowly and with concentration, place your other foot against the inside of the standing leg. Bring one or both hands in front of your chest, and the other hand to remain on support if needed. Remain for three to five breaths. Repeat the same on the other side.

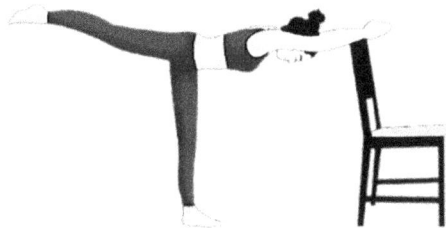

Stand behind the chair, and bring your hands onto the back of it. Come into a half fold. Start to hinge forward from your hips. Softly bend your knees but ground through the left leg. Slowly raise your right leg behind you, no higher than hip height. Keep it straight. Feel your body holding you, and use a chair as a support. Hold for three to six breaths. Repeat the opposite leg—twice on each side.

Complete your session in a chair mountain pose. Observe your breath and how you feel. Think about one thing that you're grateful for. Wigle your toes and feel the support beneath them.

HOLISTIC BALANCE — A FULL BODY JOURNEY

Today's practice embodies a holistic balance, encompassing a variety of muscle groups to ensure a comprehensive workout.

Engage in a sequence of poses that target different areas, including hamstrings, heart openers, hip openers, knees, lower back, pelvis, quadriceps, shoulders, and upper back.

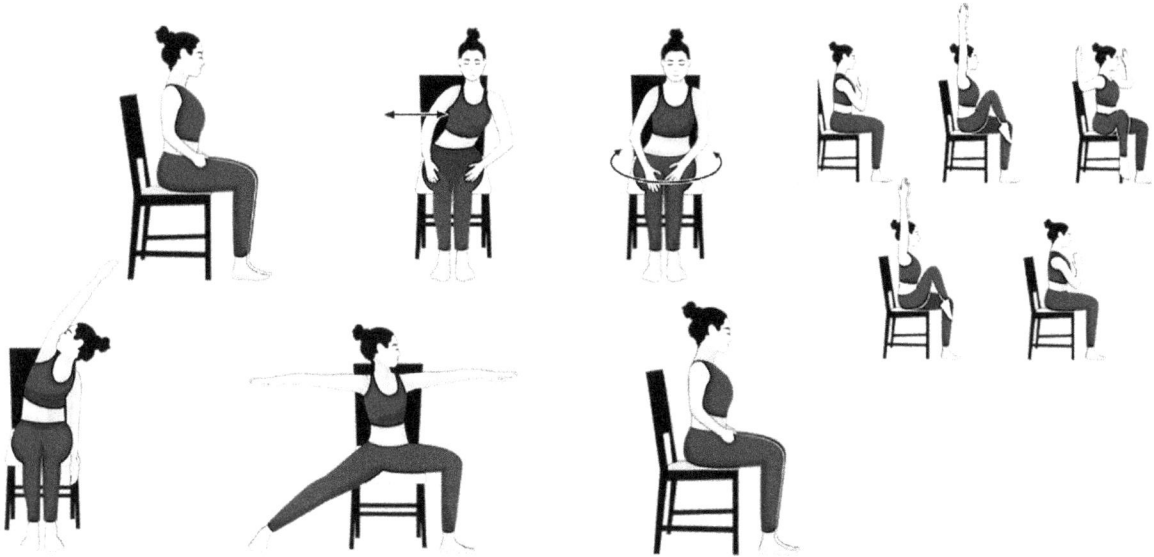

Begin in a mountain pose. You can lean to the back of the chair; however, keep your spine straight, shoulders lowered, and head above your heart. Keep your feet flat on the ground and your spine tall. Softly close your eyes or gaze downward to minimize distractions. Take a deep breath and exhale slowly. Start concentrating on your breath. Notice the sensation. Focus solely on your breath. Scan your body for any tension or discomfort, relaxing those areas with each breath. Engage your hands, moving them mindfully and feeling the sensations in your fingers and palms. Bring your focus back to your breath, following its natural flow in and out of your body. Visualize a warm, radiant light at a chosen point within your body, bringing tranquility to your entire being. Take a few more deep breaths, gradually returning your attention to the present moment. Open your eyes gently, taking a moment to appreciate the calmness and clarity you've cultivated.

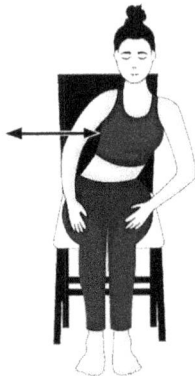

Sit with your feet hip-distance apart or together. Feel your sit bones firmly grounded to the chair. Inhale, rolling your ribs forward. Exhale and round your back, ensuring only the torso moves while your legs stay grounded. Draw circles, adjust the size as needed, and listen to your body. Repeat this movement three to five times at your own breath pace, using deep or ocean breaths. Change direction and repeat the process.

Seated Hip Circles Chair

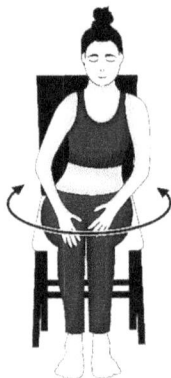

Start by placing your hands on your thighs and straightening your spine. Initiate slow circular motions with your torso, moving from the hips. Gradually increase the size of the circles as you feel comfortable. Begin the circular motion in an anticlockwise direction. Slowly reduce the size of the circles, maintaining control and awareness. Return to the center with your chin slightly tucked, bringing your focus to the rhythm of your breath.

Seated Low Lunge Pose

This easy flow will help stretch your feet, ankles, hips, and knees and strengthen your pelvic floor. Sit tall with both feet on the floor and sit bones grounded on the chair. Inhale and bend your right knee toward your chest.

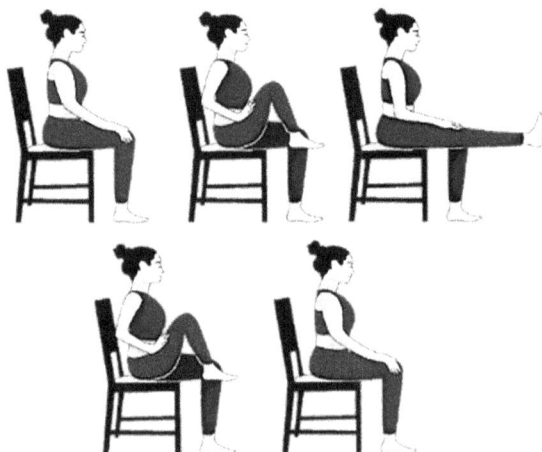

Exhale and extend your leg out. Toes up toward the ceiling. Inhale, and bring it back by bending your right knee toward your chest. Exhale, and place your foot on the floor. Repeat on the other side—a total of five times for each leg. If you need to bend your knee toward your chest, you can grab under the knee and support your move.

Chair Seated Side Stretch Pose

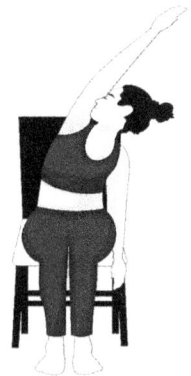

Sit upright. Place the hands on either side of the seat or your lap. Roll your shoulders down the back. Inhale and, pulling in the core, sweep the right arm above the head, creating a lateral bend on the left-hand side. Exhale into the stretch. Allow your chest and head to tilt to the left. Stay in this pose for three breaths. On the inhale, return to the center. Repeat the same with the left side.

You can choose to stay on one side for two to three breaths before switching to the other side, or you may choose to move dynamically between one side and the other on the breath. Do what feels best for your body. Repeat the same with the left side.

During the movement, you may look down at the floor, straight ahead, or up toward the top arm—please choose the option that feels right for your neck. Try to keep your mouth and jaw loose as you move.

Warrior Pose II Chair

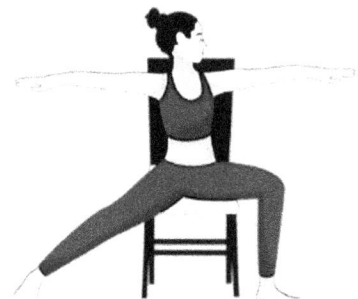

Sit on the edge of the chair. Inhale, and separate the feet. Starting on the left first, open the left leg like a goddess pose, but the left leg only. The knee aligns with the ankle and hip, forming a 90-degree angle. The foot is flat and relaxed, with the toes pointing to the left. Exhale and extend the right leg behind to make it straight in the knee. The right foot is flat here, and the toes point to the front. Make your back straight with your hands resting on the knees. Sit nice and tall. Once the body is comfortable, inhale and extend your arms at shoulder level to a nice T. Ensure the palms are face down and elbows are not bent. Finally, turn your head and gaze at your left fingers. Don't collapse; the torso is straight, and the shoulders are lowered.

While here, check the alignment of the legs—the front knee doesn't drop to the side. Stay balanced in the pose. Breathe slowly, deeply, and softly. Stay for two to three breaths.

To release the pose: Turn your head back to the center on the exhale. Lower your hands, and realign your legs to the mountain pose. Stay here for a while. Following the previous steps, counter the stretch on the other side.

NURTURING FEET, ANKLES, HIP OPENERS, AND QUADRICEPS

Today's practice is dedicated to the well-being of your feet, ankles, hip openers, and quadriceps.

Engage in stretches that promote flexibility and comfort in your feet and ankles, which is essential for maintaining a strong foundation. Embrace hip openers that encourage fluidity in your hip joints and alleviate tension, promoting ease of movement. Strengthen and stretch your quadriceps for enhanced leg functionality and overall mobility.

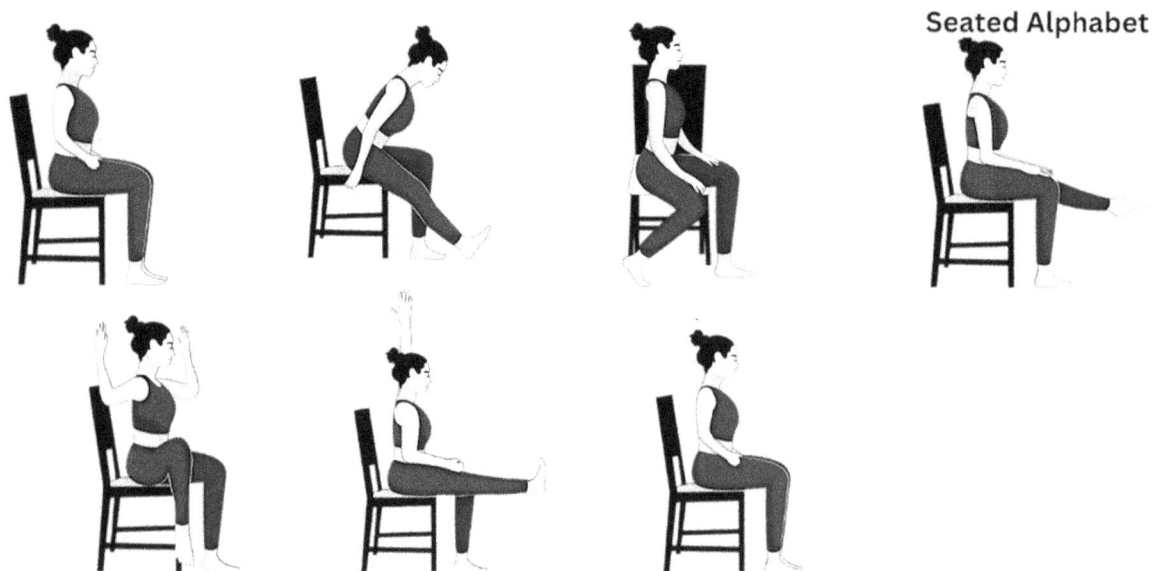

Seated Alphabet

Half Seated Forward Bend Pose Chair

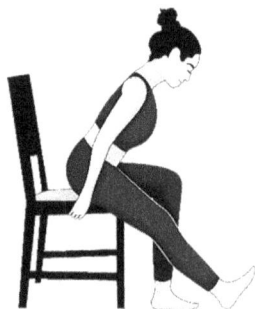

Take a deep, cleansing breath, sitting in a mountain pose. Inhale deeply through your nose, and exhale slowly through your mouth, releasing any tension or stress. Let go of the outside world for now and focus on the present moment as we embark on a journey of relaxation and rejuvenation through gentle movements and breath. Become aware of your surroundings. While seated on the chair, move your thighs forward and extend your right leg, placing the foot out, and resting it on the heels.

Point your toes upward, and press the heels firmly to stretch the sole of your foot. Take a moment to feel the sensation of the stretch in the inner sole, and remain in this position, breathing deeply for about six breaths. Focus on extending the quads, hamstrings, and calves, feeling release and relaxation in those areas.

Now, repeat the same sequence with the other leg. Pay attention to the leg with more issues, and try to hold that stretch a bit longer. You can repeat this stretching process multiple times to work on the tendons and tissues around the plantar fascia (ligament) effectively while seated in the half-seated forward bend pose on the chair. After completing both legs, take a moment to relax and settle into your seated position.

After completing both legs, release the stretch and sit back, resting your feet on the floor. Take a moment to relax and settle into your seated position.

Seated Plantar Fascia Stretch Chair

Scoot forward in the chair without going too close to the edge. Keep your right foot planted on the floor, dropping your left knee. Move your left foot underneath you or to the side, toes on the floor, as if standing on tiptoes. Gently push your knee down, stretching your toes and the bottom of your foot. Hold for a few breaths (3–5 breaths).

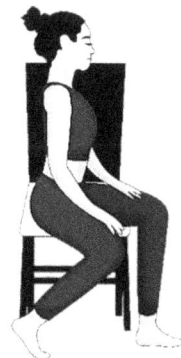

Slide your left leg straight in front, foot flat on the floor. On an out-breath, lift your foot a couple of inches off the floor. While breathing normally, make ankle circles in each direction for a few breaths. Place your foot back on the floor and slide it next to your right foot. Repeat it on another side.

Ankle Alphabet

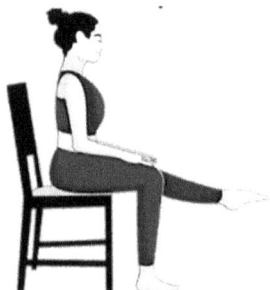

Start from the mountain pose with your feet touching the floor. Straighten your right leg in front of you with your toes pointing forward. Extend your left leg with your toes pointed toward the ceiling. Imagine that you're using your big toe to write alphabet letters. Lift your leg slightly from the floor and draw the letters twice. Repeat with the other leg. Repeat twice, then switch to your other leg. Sit nice and tall in mountain pose. Lift your left foot and place it on the right thigh. Stretch your big toe up and down and to the side with your fingers. Do it ten times and all different directions and then switch the foot.

Seated External Hip Rotation Pose Cactus Arms Chair

Sit upright, ensuring your shoulders are relaxed and your spine remains straight. Feel a sense of grounding through your hips and feet. Position your arms in a cactus shape, aligning your elbows with your shoulders and stacking your wrists above your elbows. Spread your fingers wide and direct them upward. Inhale, sweep your arms to the sides while keeping your elbows bent, as shown. As you breathe in, engage your core muscles, lengthen your neck, and draw your shoulder blades down your back.

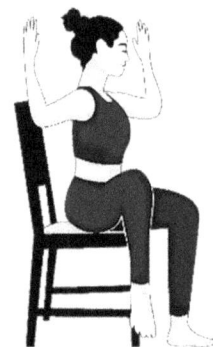

With an inhale, extend your right leg to the right side, and as you exhale, bring it back to the center. Repeat this motion eight to ten times with one leg. If your arms feel fatigued, release the cactus arm position, and take a few breaths in the mountain pose. Then, repeat the sequence on the other side.

Easy Pose Chair One Leg Opposite Arm Raised

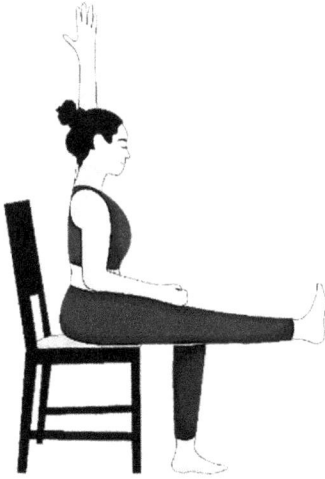

Sit nice and tall, away from the chair back. Use your ocean breath if you can.

Engage your core, and pull the belly button in toward the spine. Inhale and raise the right leg and left arm. Hold for a few breaths. Feel how your leg is activated.

Lower the leg or bend through the knee if it's too challenging. Remember to breathe and coordinate movement with breath. Release to the ground after a couple of breaths. Repeat two to three times for each side.

Day 19

BICEPS TRICEPS, ABS, AND KNEES

Today's sequence is dedicated to nurturing your shoulder arms, upper back, biceps, triceps, abs, and knees.

Engage in stretches that promote flexibility and comfort in your shoulder, arms, and upper back, releasing tension and promoting relaxation. Embrace movements targeting your biceps triceps, contributing to overall strength and stability.

Strengthen your core with poses that engage your abs, fostering stability and balance. Care for your knees with gentle stretches that support joint health and mobility.

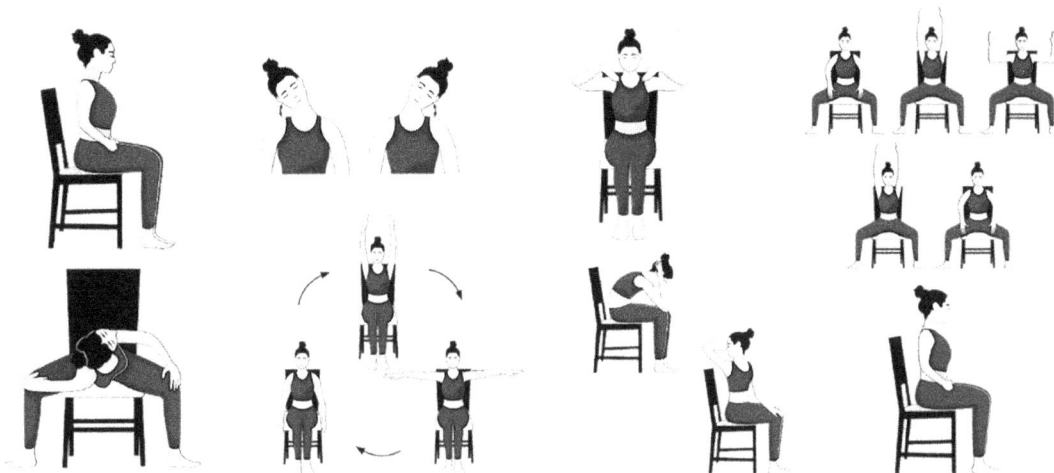

Chair Seated Shoulder Circles

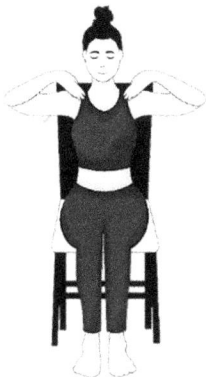

Close your eyes gently if you feel at ease, and take a few deep, cleansing breaths, engaging in abdominal breathing. Inhale deeply through your nose, allowing your abdomen to expand, and exhale slowly through your mouth, releasing any tension or stress. Let go of the outside world for now and focus on the present moment. Sit on the chair facing forward and feet hip-distance apart or together on the floor. Inhale, lift your arms to the side, parallel to the floor. Exhale, and bring fingertips to shoulders. Begin to circle in one direction. Circles can be large or small. Pause and bring attention to your breathing. Circle six to eight times in each direction. Keep your spine straight. Pause, inhale to open your arms, and lower them on the exhale, bringing them to the center.

Chair Neck Rolls

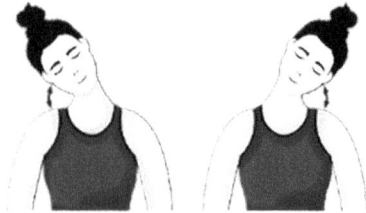

Take a couple of deep breaths.

Inhale and move your ear towards the right shoulder and exhale. Make sure that the neck is long and the shoulders are relaxed and away from the ears. On the inhale, come back to the center, exhale, and pause before switching sides. Repeat on another side, five times on both sides.

Goddess Pose on Chair Arms Flow

Inhale to rotate the hips outward, bringing the feet to 120 degrees, with toes pointing sideways and knees bent. Gently push out the inner thighs as you plant both feet firmly on the floor. Raise your arms overhead—palms facing each other—keeping shoulders away from ears. Exhale while bending elbows so that forearms are perpendicular and palms are facing forward

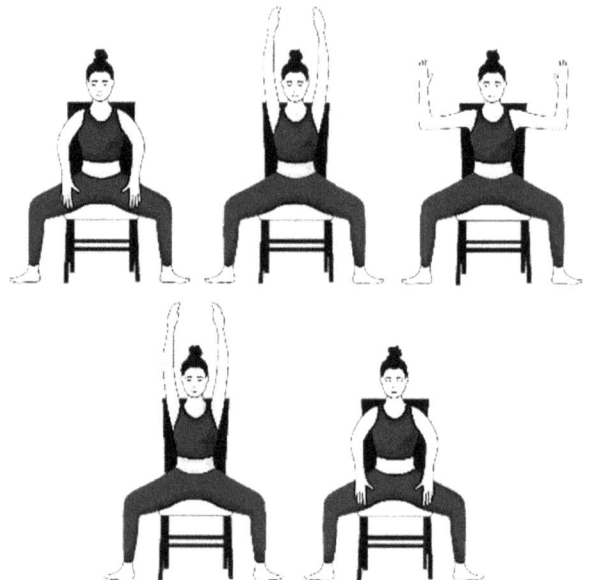

(cactus arms). Hold for thirty seconds before inhaling to extend arms up again with palms together. Lower arms back down at shoulder level in an exhale, and place hands on inner thighs before inhaling again to raise them. Complete four to six repetitions of this flow, coordinating breathing as needed, then release and relax. Once you complete it, remain in the goddess pose for your next pose.

Revolved Goddess Pose

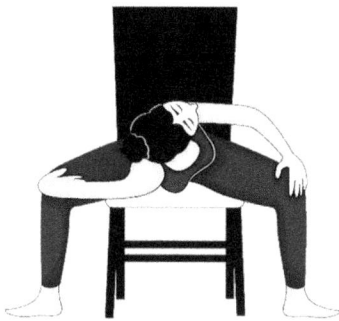

Sit up nice and tall. Pull shoulders away from the ears, shoulder blades going down the back. Check that your knees align with the hips and ankles, forming a 90-degree angle. Place your hand on the thighs. Bring your heels slightly in, and turn the toes slightly out. Roll the shoulders back. Inhale, place your hands on the knees, and slowly bend forward on the exhale, with your back parallel to the ground. Twist to the left first, inhale, and draw the navel into the spine. While exhaling, twist the torso to the left. Take the left shoulder back and the right forward.

Stay here for three to six breaths or as long as comfortable, twisting your neck to fix your gaze over the shoulder. To release, inhale, release the twist and forward bend, and return to the center. Take a few breaths, and as you're ready, exhale and, this time, twist and turn to another side. Bring the right shoulder back and the left forward.

Chair Mountain Pose Sweeping Arms Flow

This will help you to warm up your shoulders. Sit in a mountain pose. Inhale reaching the arms up, palms facing each other above your head. Exhale and slowly release them down, palms facing down. Inhale reaching the arms up; exhale palms face down. Repeat the sequence for another two or three times.

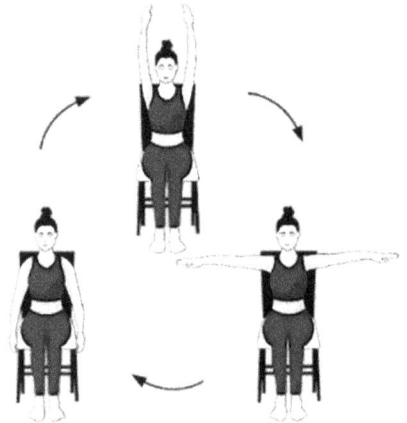

Seated Chair One Hand behind Head Elbow Knee Flow

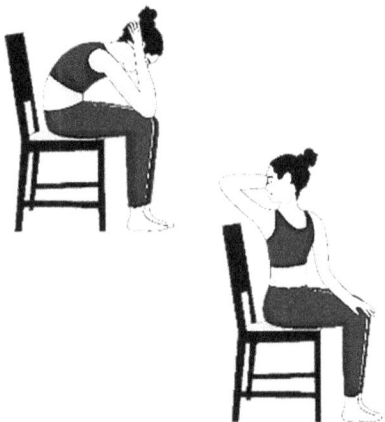

Place your palms with elbows bent at the back of your head. On the exhale, bend forward at the hips, bringing your elbows together, and lean on your knees with your elbows. On the inhale, sit up straight and leave your left arm resting on the thighs. At the same time, bring your right elbow back and look over that elbow. On the exhale, bend forward again, bringing your elbows together.

Inhale—sit up straight once more while bringing your left elbow back and looking over that elbow. Repeat this sequence, coordinating your breath with the movements three to five times.

HIP OPENERS, PSOAS MUSCLE, HAMSTRINGS, ABS, AND LOWER BACK HARMONY

Welcome to Day 20 of your chair yoga journey! Today's practice is about cultivating harmony within your hip openers, psoas muscles, hamstrings, abs, and lower back.

Engage in hip-opening stretches that encourage fluidity and release tension in your hips. Pay special attention to your pelvic muscle, which connects your upper and lower body. Stretch your hamstrings for enhanced lower body flexibility.

Strengthen your core with poses that engage your abs, fostering stability and balance. Address your lower back with gentle stretches, promoting comfort and relaxation.

Embrace this opportunity to nurture these essential muscle groups, fostering a harmonious connection between body and mind.

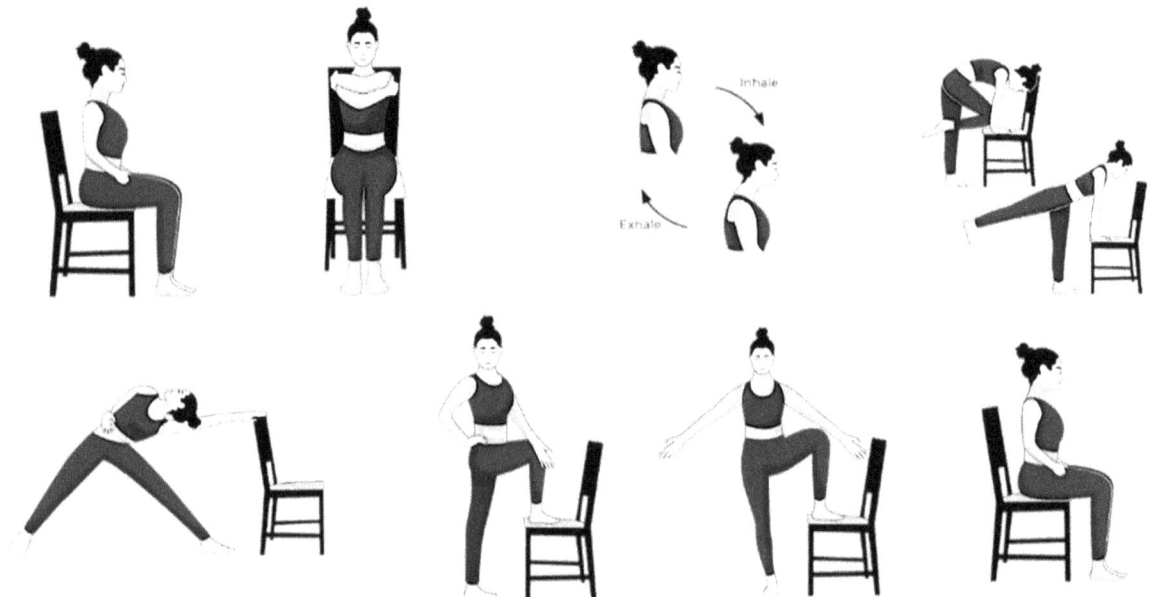

Bear Hug Stretch Pose

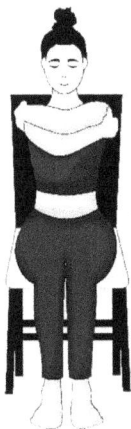

Start by sitting in mountain pose getting ready. Take a few deep breaths.

The hug will help to stretch your upper back and shoulders. On the inhale, hug yourself. Hold on to your shoulders as you open up your upper back while keeping your spine and back straight. Take a couple of deep breaths

Turtle Neck Flow

This movement lengthens and strengthens the neck muscles. The neck muscles are connected to the shoulders and back of the thoracic spine. This movement stretches those muscles.

On the inhale, take the chin forward, going beyond the chest and collarbone. Exhale to come back to the center. Repeat it three to six times, making sure the extension is more with each round without moving the shoulders. Don't rush, as the slower you go, the better the sensation of the deeper stretch in tissues of the neck and shoulders.

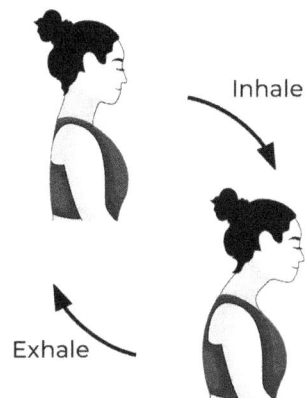

Standing Table Top Pose With Knee To Nose Flow Chair

Begin by standing tall and upright, squarely facing the chair seat. Inhale deeply, allowing the breath to steady you. On the exhale, gently place your hands on the chair, creating a supportive connection, envisioning your neck as an extension of your spine. Continue exhaling as you lengthen your spine and direct the extension through your head. Glide your right leg behind you to its fullest extent. As you exhale, draw the right knee toward your nose, curving it inward. Inhale again, send the leg back by extending it, creating length, and then exhale to bring the knee toward your nose again. Repeat this fluid sequence three to six times on one side. Return to your stance in the mountain pose, taking a moment to stand firmly and breathe. Mirror the sequence on the opposite side, maintaining your focus and intention throughout.

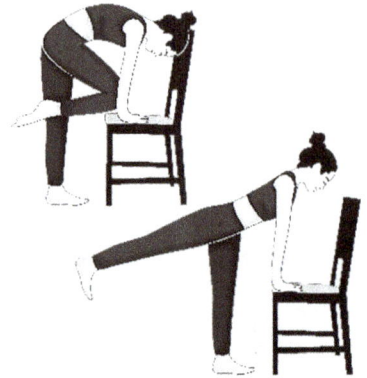

Triangle Pose Chair

Position yourself about an arm's length behind the chair. Place the chair to your left at arm's distance and gently rest your left hand on it. Inhale as you extend your arm, ensuring your left foot forms a 90-degree angle and the right foot turns slightly inward at 45 degrees. Hold this posture for approximately four to eight breaths before transitioning to the other side.

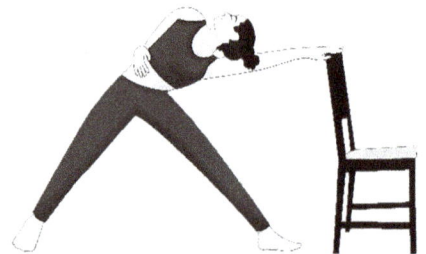

Standing Twist Chair

Stand in front of the chair and place your right foot on it, forming a 90-degree angle. Ensure your left standing leg aligns with your hip, toes forward, and knee gently unlocked. Let your left hand rest on the outside of your right knee, and place your right hand on your lower back. On the inhale, elongate your spine upward. On the exhale, engage in a gentle twist toward your bent knee, spiraling your ribs and spine to the right. Hold for three to six breaths. Release, relax, and repeat this sequence on the opposite side.

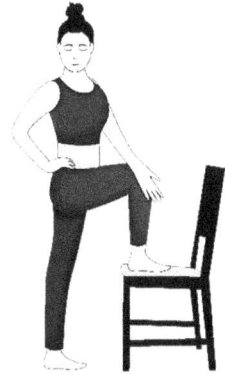

Tree Pose Chair

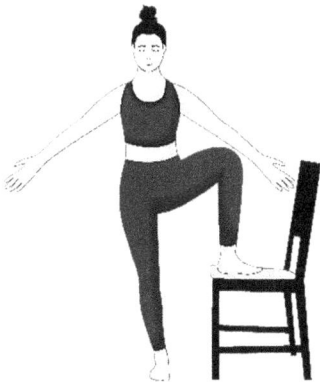

Starting from standing, ground your left foot firmly, and position your right foot onto the chair's seat. Use your right hand on the chair's back for balance if needed. Check your right knee—ensure visibility of your toes/foot. Adjust for a comfortable 90-degree angle, sparing your knee undue strain and enhancing alignment. Extend your arms like an inverted V, fix your gaze ahead, engage your core, and activate your glutes. Inhale deeply, and if comfortable, gently close your eyes. Exhale fully, bringing your right foot down to meet your left on the floor. Let your hands rest by your sides, palms forward. Mirror this sequence on the left side. Continue for two deep breaths on each side.

Once you finish, sit down in a comfortable seated position in the center of the chair, leaving some space between the back of the chair and your back. Rock back and forth until you locate your sit bones. Keep your feet hip-distance apart and flat on the floor. If you prefer, bring your knees together. Close your eyes or soften your gaze. Bring your attention to your breath, feeling the rise and fall of your chest and the expansion and contraction of your abdomen. Inhale deeply in and out. Inhale while counting to four, hold your breath for four, and exhale, counting to six. If these intervals are too long, do three, three, and four. Continue this rhythmic breathing for two minutes, allowing your body and mind to relax.

GENTLE RESTORATION — NECK, BICEPS, HIPS, AND KNEES

Today's practice is a gentle restoration day, focusing on your neck, biceps, hips, and knees. Take this opportunity to give your body a chance to rest and rejuvenate.

Engage in stretches that provide comfort and release tension in your neck, promoting relaxation. Embrace gentle movements that target your biceps, stimulating circulation and flexibility.

Address your hips and knees with mild stretches, encouraging mobility and joint health. Allow yourself to move through each pose with ease, appreciating the refreshing nature of this practice.

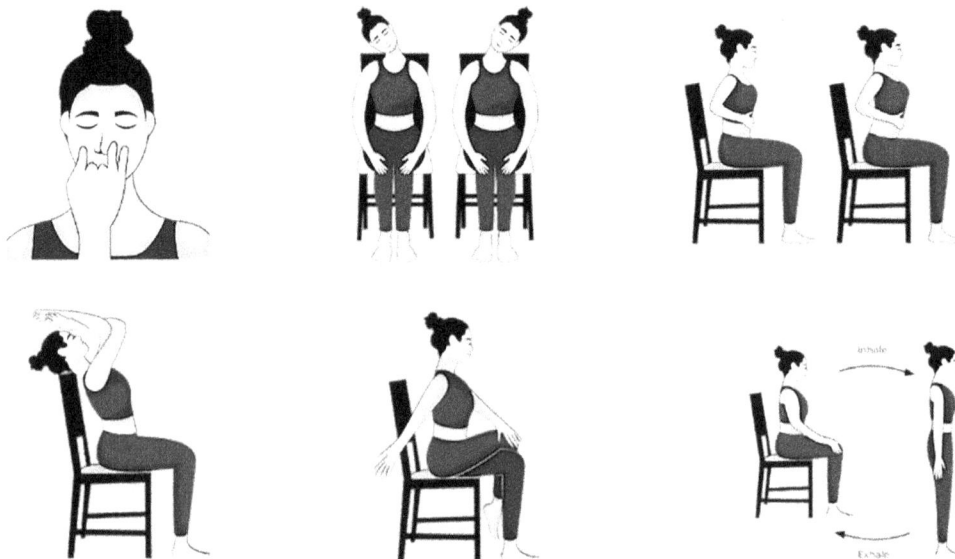

Alternate Nostril Breathing Chair

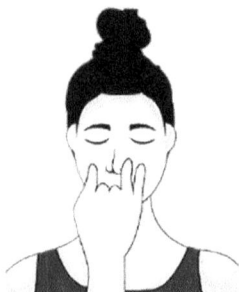

Sit nice and tall in a mountain pose. Rest your left hand on your left thigh or in your lap or use it to support the elbow of your right arm. Close your right nostril with the thumb of that hand, inhale through the left, and then close it off with your ring finger and pinky. Exhale through the right nostril for a short pause before repeating this cycle three to five times with both nostrils. When finished, return to regular breathing.

Chair Neck Rolls

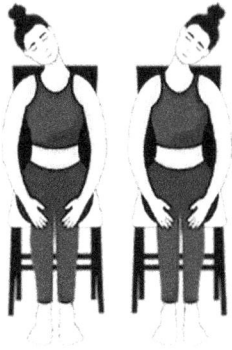

Return to the mountain pose. Find your center, and take a few relaxed breaths. Inhale, elongate your spine, and feel your sit bones grounding while envisioning the crown of your head reaching upward. Tuck your chin slightly. Inhale, and turn your head to the right, then exhale. Inhale back to center, exhale, and pause before switching sides. Repeat on the other side. Complete this sequence two—four times on each side.

Seated Pelvic Tilt Tuck

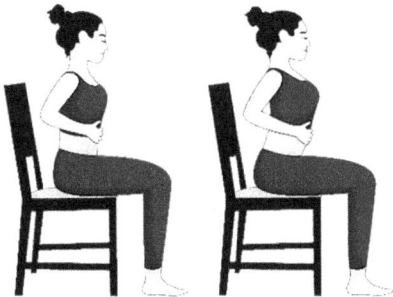

Place feet firmly on the floor in mountain pose, arms resting on your knees, spine erect. Place your hands on top of the pelvis crest to feel the movement. This is a slight movement, just tilting the tailbone back and forth. Inhale as you tilt the pelvis forward, like tipping a bowl full of water ahead. Exhale as you tilt the pelvis backward. Repeat for six to eight cycles.

Seated Backbend with Eagle Arms In Chair

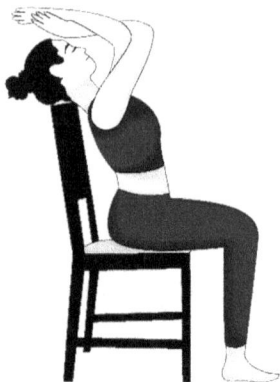

Sit up nice and tall. Commence by sliding your right arm beneath the left, attempting to cross at the elbows. Either clasp your palms or meet the backs of your hands. Elevate your elbows to shoulder height, then guide your forearms outward from your face. Ensure a firm grip as you lift, sensing your shoulders broaden. Maintain steady breathing for a few cycles. You can gently arch your upper back and raise your elbows if comfortable. Switch sides. Remain in the position for 3–4 breaths.

Seated with Eagle Legs Pose Chair Variation

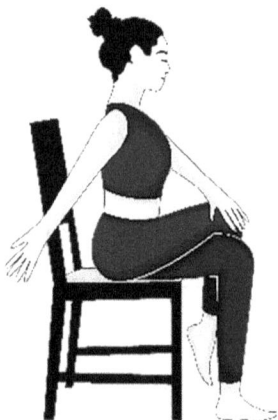

Gently place your right thigh over the left, and if you can, put your foot behind the left calf. Rest your left hand upon your right thigh. Stretch your right arm. Inhale and elongate your spine with each breath in. Exhale as you press the right arm into the chair's back, gently guiding your right thigh with your left hand—within your comfortable range. You don't need to stay in the pose if you cannot at this stage. You can move in and out of it slowly, changing sides. Repeat five times on each side. Or you can remain in the pose for three to five deep breaths and switch sides.

Chair Mountain Pose Standing Flow

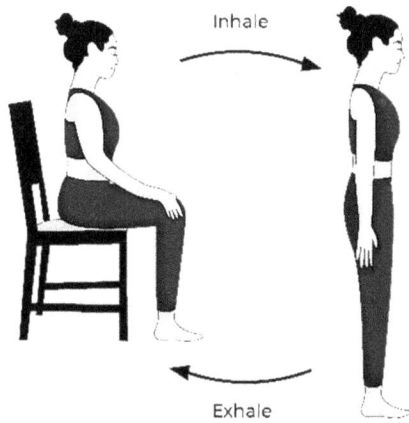

This is a simple-looking but powerful short sequence to develop strength in the lower body. Engage your thighs and glutes, and on the inhale, stand up, and slowly, on the exhale, sit down. Repeat five times. If you need a challenge, slow down when sitting down—feel your quads and hamstrings in action.

HAMSTRINGS, ABS, KNEES, SHOULDERS, AND GLUTEUS STRENGTH

Today's chair yoga routine is dedicated to strengthening your hamstrings, abs, knees, shoulders, and gluteus muscles. Through a series of purposeful poses, you'll engage these muscle groups for enhanced well-being.

Stretch and activate your hamstrings for improved lower body flexibility. Strengthen your core with poses that engage your abs, fostering stability and balance. Care for your knees and shoulders with gentle stretches that support joint health and mobility.

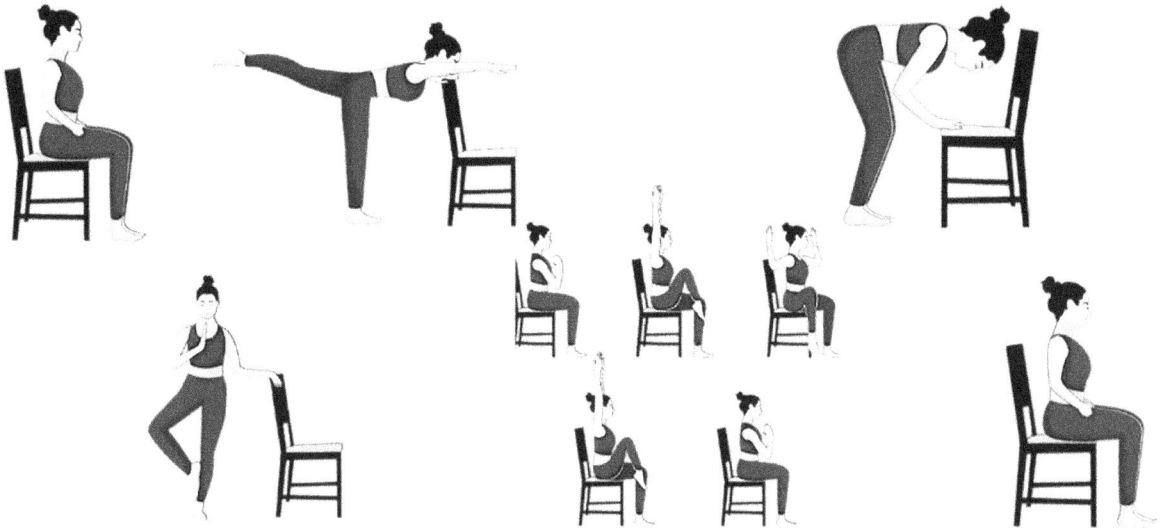

Let's begin in a chair mountain pose. You will perform a so-called "box breathing." It's ratioed breathing that uses a set length of inhalation, breath holds, and exhalations—inhaled and exhaled through the nose. At your own comfortable pace, start to slow and deepen your breathing to a point where you are still breathing easily and without losing your breath. Inhale for four seconds and hold the breath for four seconds. Exhale for four seconds and hold the breath out for seconds. Repeat for three to four times or as much as you need.

Warrior Pose on the Chair

Stand in front of the chair and place both hands on the back. Breathe in, and slowly shift your weight onto your left leg. Extend your right one behind you with your toes touching the floor. Once you find your balance, slowly tip your body forward, raising your right leg and simultaneously raising your left arm. Stay if it's too challenging, then keep both arms on the chair's back. Or raise the arm, but don't fully lift your right leg. Let the tips of the toes touch the floor. Remain in the pose for three to four breaths and switch sides. Focus on your breath.

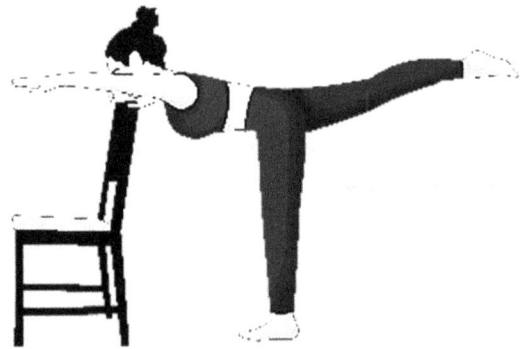

Standing Push-Ups Pose Chair

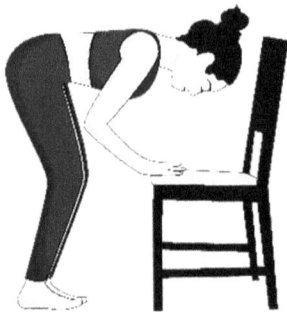

Stand in front of the chair. On the inhale, feel how your spine is lengthening. Bend your knees slightly, and bend at the hip crease on your arms. Arms are under your shoulders, slightly bent through the elbows. Lengthen your spine and neck. Move dynamically in and out as doing push-ups. Bend the elbows, allowing the chest to come closer to the chair. Straighten the arms by pushing into the chair. Repeat five times.

Tree Pose Holding onto Chair

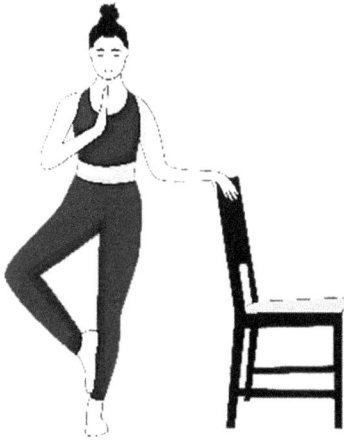

Stand next to the chair. Find a steady point to gaze at in front of you. Move your weight to the leg closest to the support. Square hips to the front, and keep them even with the floor. Place your other foot against the inside of the standing leg—keeping your toes on the floor, calf, or above the knee. Whatever feels right to you. Press the bent knee out gently. Bring one or both hands in front of your chest. Keep one arm on the back of the chair for support if needed. Take three to five breaths and repeat with the opposite side.

Seated Low Lunge Variation Chair Arms Raised Flow

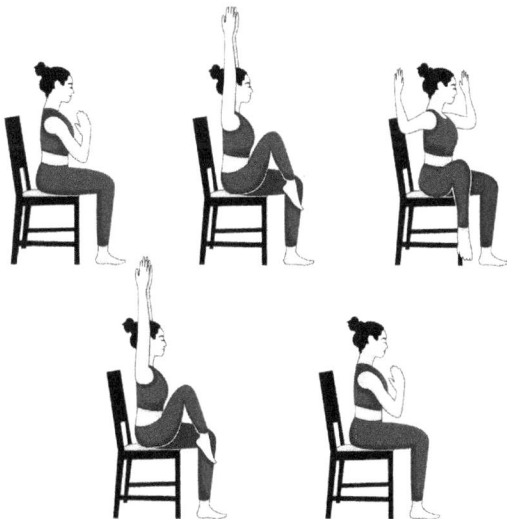

Sit up nice and tall in a mountain position. On the inhale, reach your arms and right knee up together. On the exhale, open your arms to a cactus—arms bend at the elbows at the shoulder level. Simultaneously, bring your right knee to the side. Inhale, and reach both arms back up toward the sky, lifting your knee toward your chest at a center. Exhale, and put your right knee down, returning your arms to the prayer position. Repeat on the other side. Repeat it twice on each side. If you need a challenge—repeat it three times.

COMPREHENSIVE RENEWAL ROUTINE

The most challenging part is done—you've shown up. Today's practice is a comprehensive renewal encompassing various muscle groups for a refreshing experience.

Engage in stretches to refresh your feet and ankles, promoting comfort and support. Embrace poses that enhance your hamstrings' flexibility and strength. Experience fluidity in your hip joints through hip openers.

Address your knees, lower back, and pelvic muscles with targeted stretches, promoting joint health and alleviating tension. Strengthen your shoulders and arms while addressing upper back discomfort.

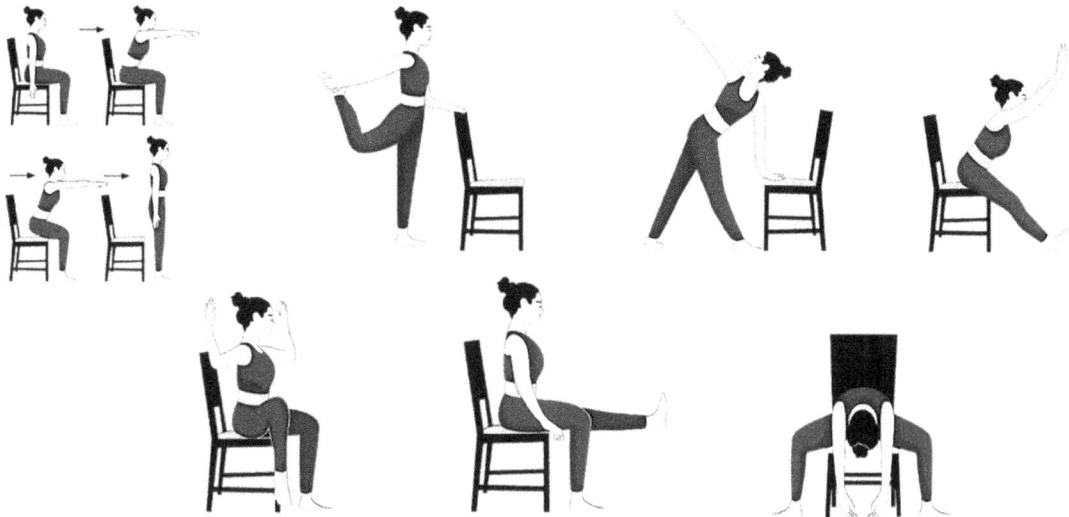

Chair Mountain Pose Stand-Up Flow

Start in a mountain pose. The spine is nice and tall, shoulders rolled back. Take a few breaths and concentrate on coordinating your breath with a movement. Reach your arms forward to help you lift your hips off the chair. Hold this position for a couple of breaths and stand up. Feel the ground under your feet. Sit back down with your arms next to you. Repeat five more times.

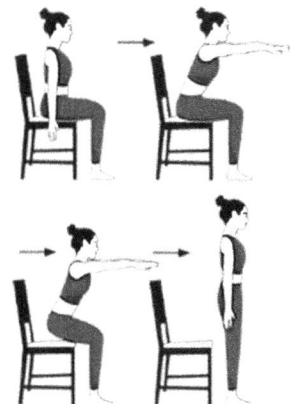

Dancer Pose with Chair

Stand with feet hip-width apart. Engage the core, roll your shoulders back, keep your head neutral, and relax your jaw. Shift weight to the left leg, inhale, and sweep the right arm backward.

Bend right knee, and grip right foot's instep. Engage the glutes and lift the leg behind, creating traction to open the shoulder. Ensure a moderately bent knee and engage the core for lower back support. Hold, breathe, exhale to stand, then repeat the other side. Hold for three to six breaths.

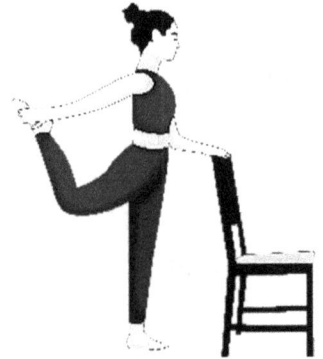

Revolved Triangle Pose with Chair

Stand, facing the seat of a chair. Step the left foot back. Keep the right foot pointing toward the chair. Turn the left foot out, toes pointing to the left, creating a 90-degree angle between the right and left foot. Take the right hand to the seat of the chair. Rest the left hand on the left hip or reach the left arm to the sky. Hold for three breaths. Bend the right knee and push through the feet with a steady core to release the pose. Repeat it on another side.

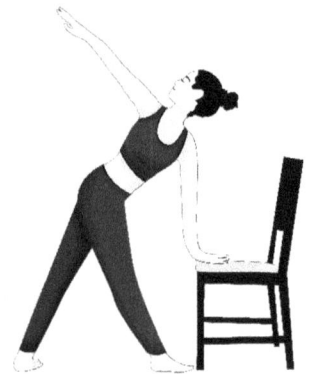

Seated Downward Facing Dog Pose Chair

Extend the legs—one at a time. On the inhale, flex the feet toward yourself. Extend the arms up, exhale to lean forward slightly from the hips, hugging the navel in. Think of keeping your back flat. Scoot the sit bones back to help balance. Keep the neck long. Bend your knees slightly if needed. Stay in this position for a few breaths. If required, take a break and repeat it. If this pose is not available, with both legs stretched out, then alternate legs. Pay attention to the leg with more issues, and try to hold that stretch a bit longer. After completing both legs, release the stretch, and sit back, resting your feet on the floor.

Seated External Hip Rotation Pose Cactus Arms Chair

Sit upright, ensuring your shoulders are relaxed and your spine remains straight. Feel a sense of grounding through your hips and feet. Position your arms in a cactus shape, aligning your elbows with your shoulders and stacking your wrists above your elbows. Spread your fingers wide and direct them upward. Inhale, sweep your arms to the sides while keeping your elbows bent, as shown. As you breathe in, engage your core muscles, lengthen your neck, and draw your shoulder blades down your back. With an inhale, extend your right leg to the right side, and as you exhale, bring it back to the center. Repeat this motion eight to ten times with one leg. If your arms feel fatigued, release the cactus arm position, and take a few breaths in the mountain pose. Then, repeat the sequence on the other side.

Easy Pose Chair One Leg Opposite Arm Raised

Sit nice and tall, away from the chair back. Use your ocean breath if you can.

Engage your core, and pull the belly button in toward the spine. Inhale and raise the right leg and left arm. Hold for a few breaths. Feel how your leg is activated. Lower the leg or bend through the knee if it's too challenging. Remember to breathe and coordinate movement with breath. Release to the ground after a couple of breaths. Repeat two to three times for each side.

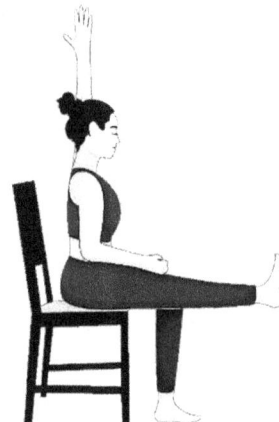

Wide Legged Forward Bend Pose Chair Hands Floor

Open legs wide, keeping knees and toes in the same direction. Stack your knees over your ankles. Ground through all four corners of feet. Inhale and raise arms overhead. On the exhale, fold forward. Listen to your body, and go as low as your body lets you. It doesn't matter if it's only a few inches. You can use blocks or a stack of books to bring the floor closer to you. Stay here for three deep breaths. If you're comfortable—remain for longer.

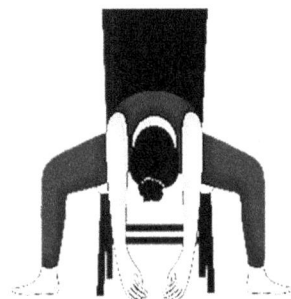

Day 24

COMPREHENSIVE MUSCLE FOCUS

Welcome to Day 24 of your chair yoga journey! Today's practice offers a comprehensive approach, engaging various muscle groups for a well-rounded experience.

This session directs attention to the abs, hamstrings, heart openers, hip openers, knees, lower back, pelvic muscles, quadriceps, and gluteus. Embrace this opportunity to nurture essential muscle groups, fostering a harmonious connection between body and mind.

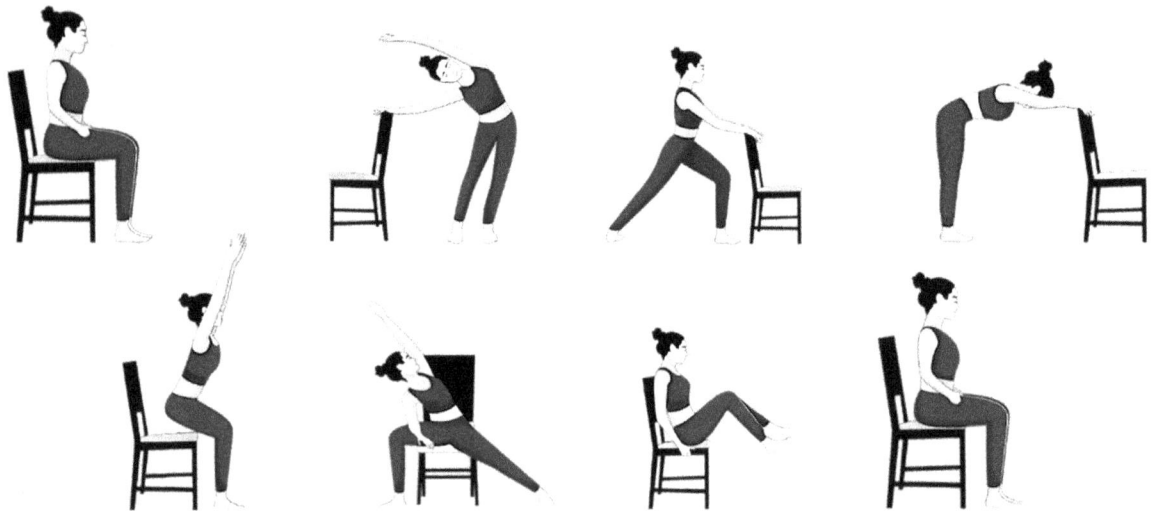

Begin in a mountain pose. You can lean to the back of the chair; however, keep your spine straight and shoulders lowered. Keep your feet flat on the ground and your spine tall. Softly close your eyes or gaze downward to minimize distractions. Take a deep breath and exhale slowly. Start concentrating on your breath. Notice the sensation. Focus solely on your breath. Scan your body for any tension or discomfort, relaxing those areas with each breath. Engage your hands, moving them mindfully and feeling the sensations in your fingers and palms. Bring your focus back to your breath, following its natural flow in and out of your body.

Standing Lateral Side Bend Flexion Chair

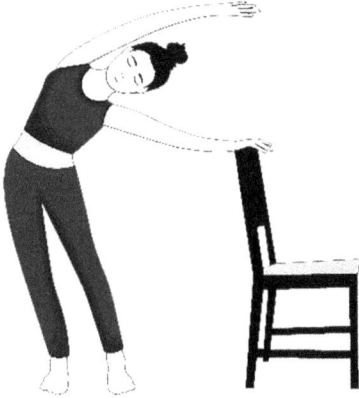

Plant left palm on the back of the chair. Stretch it out, and stand with your back straight and shoulders lowered. On the inhale, raise your right arm overhead.

Exhale and lean toward the left. Look toward your upper arm or look straight in front of you. Feel the lateral stretch. Stay in this position for three to five breaths. If this is too challenging, repeat five times on each side going into and out of the stretch.

Warrior Pose I with Chair in Front

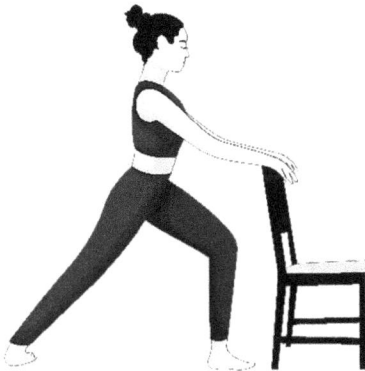

Step your right foot forward, bending the knee and keeping the knee in line with the ankle. Turn your foot at a 45-degree angle, flat on the floor. Square the hips. Keeping the back leg strong and straight, feeling both legs stretched and stable with the chest lifted. Hips are parallel to the shoulders. Remain in the position for three breaths. Repeat the same on the other side. Repeat each side twice.

Standing Forward Bend Chair

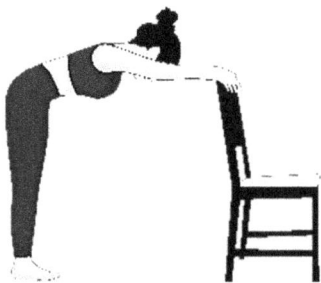

Stand behind the chair. Engage kneecaps by lifting them upward, cultivating height in your stance. Rest both arms on the chair's back. Begin a gentle step back with both legs, finding a comfortable stretch. Raise your arms toward the ceiling, palms forward. Experience a full-body stretch. Take a few deep breaths, and hinge from your waist on the exhale, keeping the legs straight. Distribute your weight between feet. Extend your arms and place palms atop a chair about three feet ahead. Press palms gently, avoiding weight transfer. Sustain length through the back, elongating the spine parallel to the floor.

Chair Pose Hovering Above Chair

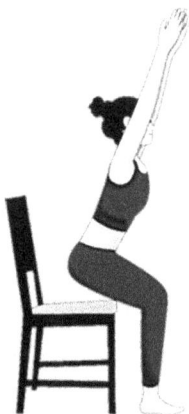

Maintain an upright posture, and lift your arms above your head while exhaling deeply. Inhale and move into a chair pose, gently raising yourself on your feet above the chair. Inhale through your nose, and exhale audibly through your mouth.

Exhale and return to a seated position, arms still extended overhead. Inhale again and resume the chair pose. Repeat this sequence three to six times.

Extended Side Angle Pose Variation Elbow Arm Chair

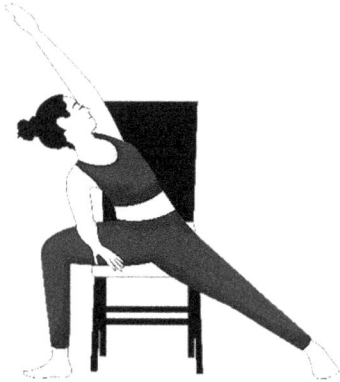

Inhale and turn your right foot outward, placing the right thigh on the chair.

Exhale, extending your left leg to the left side of the chair while lifting your right arm and stretching the side as you gaze upward. Hold the pose for three breaths, inhaling and exhaling deeply. Repeat on the other side.

Boat Pose Variation on Chair

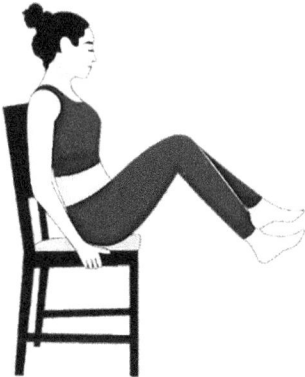

Sit straight and, on the inhale, grab the sides of the chair with your hands, positioning them right behind your buttocks. Curl your four fingers underneath the chair while resting your thumbs near the buttocks. Your weight should be on the outer edges of your palms. As you exhale, lift your feet off the floor while keeping your knees bent. Squeeze your inner thighs to keep your legs together, and cross your ankles, aligning them with the chair seat. Inhale and lengthen your spine as you engage your core, and draw your abdomen to bear the weight of your legs. You'll naturally lean back, maintaining an open chest while using your hands on the chair for balance and reducing pressure on the lower back. Stay in this position for three to four breaths, rest, and repeat it again.

Before you proceed with your day, take a moment to savor the positive energy you've cultivated during this session. Feel the chair beneath you, anchoring you in the present moment. Turn your attention inward with your eyes gently closed or a soft gaze. Tune in to the gentle rhythm of your breath. Release any lingering tension or stress with each breath out, allowing a profound sense of relaxation to wash over you, like a soothing wave caressing the shore. Pause to express gratitude for the dedicated time you've invested in your well-being. Recognize the enduring peace that resides within you, accessible through chair yoga. Now, as you gently open your eyes, carry this newfound serenity with you as you prepare to transition to the next phase with revitalized energy and heightened mindfulness.

Day 25

MUSCLE ACTIVATION

Welcome to Day 25 of your chair yoga journey! If you're reading this, congratulations—your commitment is truly admirable. You've come a long way on this path to wellness and mindfulness.

Embrace poses that activate your knees, encouraging joint health and mobility. Cultivate fluidity in your hip joints through hip openers, enhancing your overall movement. Stretch your hamstrings, promoting flexibility and lower body strength.

Embrace this opportunity to nurture these essential muscle groups, fostering a harmonious connection between body and mind as you work toward your goals.

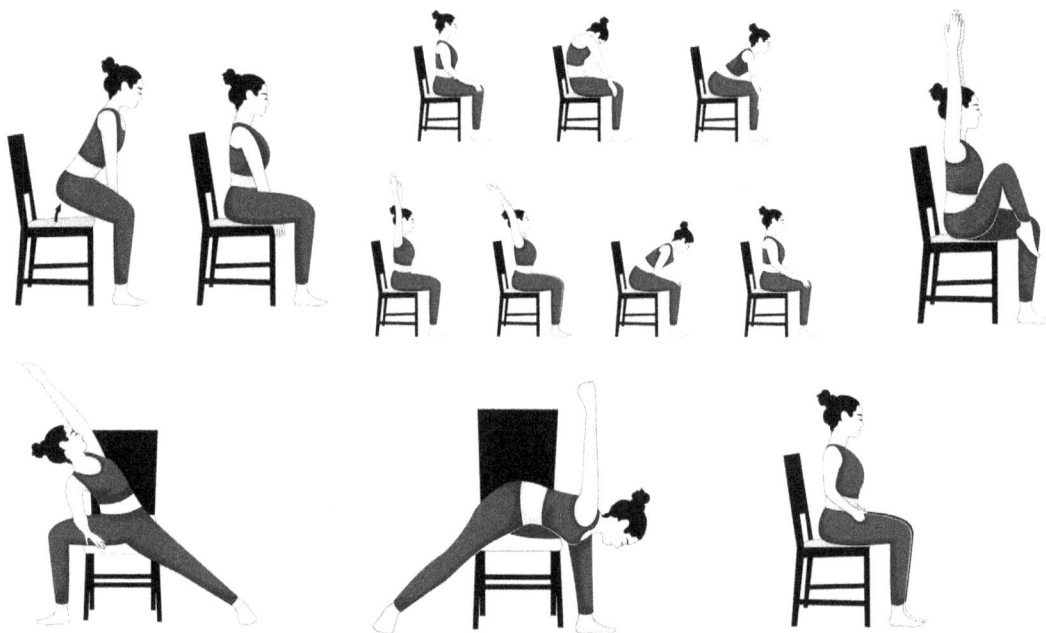

Easy Pose Chair to Chair Pose Flow

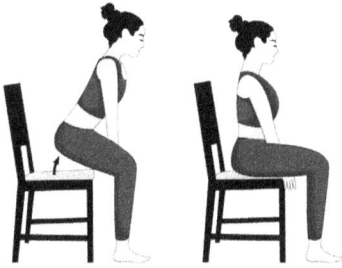

Sit tall, feet flat on the floor, hands on your lap. Take a few breaths to calm your breath, and concentrate on it. Think of the breath and movement coordination. Inhale, lean forward and activate glutes and quads. Lift hips, knees slightly bent. Look ahead, hands on knees. Exhale as you lower yourself to a seated position.Repeat three to five times.

Seated Half Forward Fold Pose Chair Flow

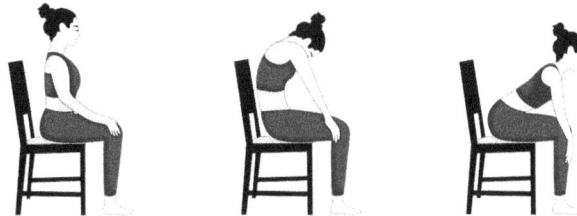

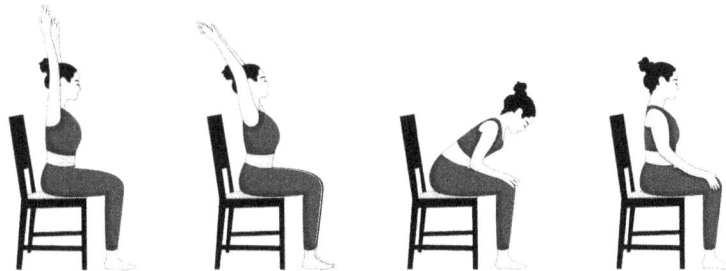

Sit comfortably in a chair, spine tall, and feel grounded on the floor. On the inhale, round your spine, and on the exhale, lean forward. Allow your hands to hold onto your knees, and lean back, arching your back. Inhale, and raise your arms above your head. And if you feel comfortable, slightly lean back. On the exhale, fold over your thighs. Come back to the neutral position. Repeat the sequence two more times. Work with a breath.

Seated Low Lunge Variation Chair Arms Raised

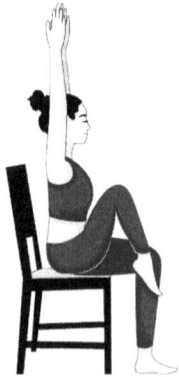

Sit tall with the spine extended. Engage your core. Notice all the muscles that take part in it when you cough. Engage the core with the belly button pulled in. Raise both your arms, and lift one leg and lower. Repeat the opposite side. Repeat three to six times for each leg.

Extended Side Angle Pose Variation Elbow Arm Chair

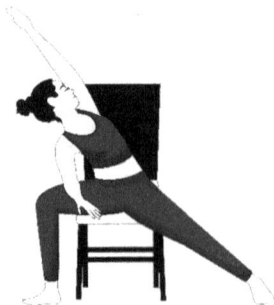

Inhale and turn your right foot outward, placing the right thigh on the chair.

Exhale, extend your left leg to the left side of the chair while lifting your right arm and stretching the side as you gaze upward. Hold the pose for three breaths, inhaling and exhaling deeply. Repeat on the other side.

Humble Warrior Pose Chair

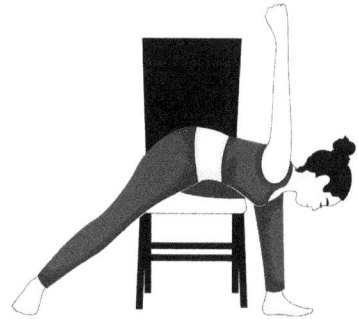

Turn your body to the left with your left leg bent over the chair seat. Place the left leg in an "L" shape. The right leg is stretched out behind you to the right side of the chair, with the foot flat and relaxed and the toes pointing to the front. Extend the spine upward, pulling the belly in and lifting the pelvic floor. Gently interlace your fingers behind your back. Inhale, and expand your chest. And as you exhale, firmly press all four corners of the feet toward the ground. Take another deep breath, pull the arms behind you, and turn the chest and shoulders toward the left side, facing the left foot. As you exhale, bend forward from the hips, gently move toward the left side, keep the chest and shoulders in a twist toward the left, extend the arms behind you upward, and bring the head toward the left foot. Do not droop the neck and head. Think about your neck and head as an extension of your spine.

To release, inhale, look up first, and lift the neck and chest. Inhale, lift the entire torso and come back to the center. With the feet still firmly grounded, release the lock of the hands. Repeat on the opposite side.

Place one hand on your belly and the other on your chest. Feel them moving with each breath in and out, a gentle reminder of the life force within you. Pay close attention to your neck, letting go of any tension accumulated during practice. Are your shoulders relaxed? Allow them to melt away any remaining stress.

Now, take a moment to reflect on how you feel. Notice the subtle changes in your body, the quieting of your mind, and the sense of inner peace that chair yoga has brought you. This is your time to unwind, to let go, and to savor the stillness within.

SUN SALUTATION ON THE CHAIR

Sun salutation variation sitting on a chair combines stretching, strengthening, and breath awareness for various benefits.

It stretches and strengthens muscles, including the spine, arms, and legs. It enhances overall flexibility and lubricates joints.

This sequence promotes conscious breath awareness, improving focus and effectiveness. It supports spinal health and corrects posture issues over time. This routine also calms the nervous system, providing relaxation and stress relief.

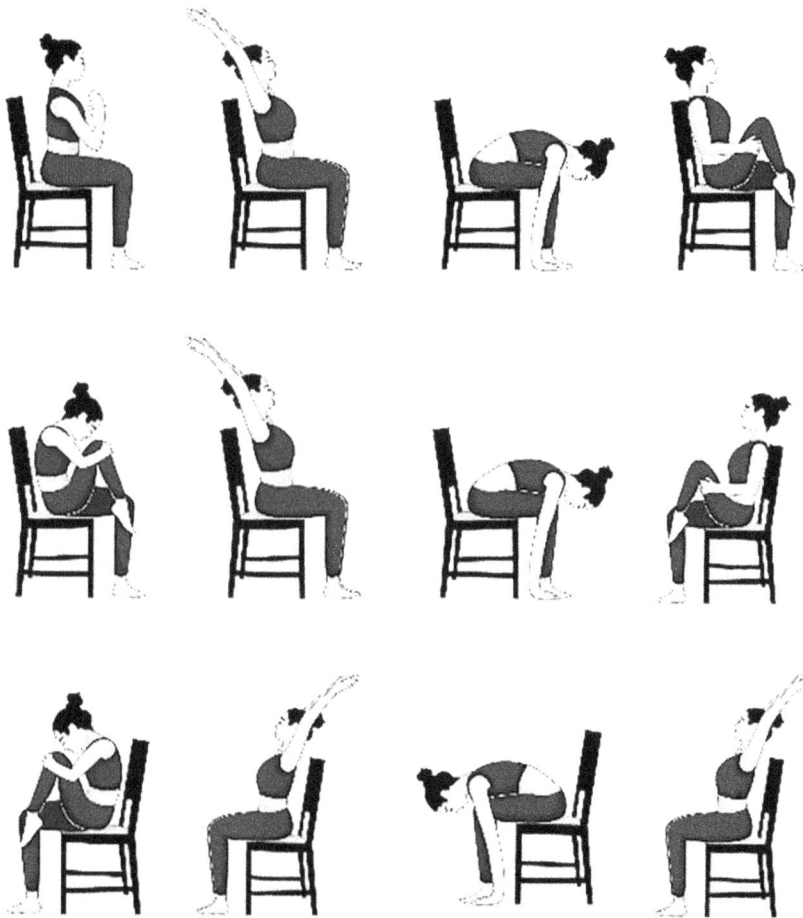

Begin in a mountain pose. You can lean to the back of the chair; however, keep your spine straight and shoulders lowered. Keep your feet flat on the ground and your spine tall. Softly close your eyes or gaze downward to minimize distractions. Take a deep breath and exhale slowly. Start concentrating on your breath. Notice the sensation. Focus solely on your breath. Scan your body for any tension or discomfort, relaxing those areas with each breath. Engage your hands, moving them mindfully and feeling the sensations in your fingers and palms. Bring your focus back to your breath, following its natural flow in and out of your body.

On the inhale, raise your arms. Feel your chest, shoulders, and arms stretching. If you feel comfortable, slightly tilt back. With the exhale from the hips, go forward and fold over your thighs. Stay here for one breath. Slowly come up. With the exhale, lift your right knee and hold it with your hand. Raise the knee toward you and look up. Press the thighs toward you, and bring the head toward the knee with your exhale. Release the leg and rest.

Now, with the inhale, raise the arms. Bend from the hips and fold forward. Stay down for one breath. Slowly come up. Repeat now on the other side. On the exhale, lift your left knee toward you and hold it with your hand; look up. Exhale, press the thighs toward you and bring the head toward the knee. Release the leg and rest. On the inhale, raise your arms, and with the exhale, go down by bending from the hips forward. Slowly come back to the center, and raise your arms up with the inhale. Stay for one more deep breath, and come back to a mountain pose. Repeat the sequence three times.

Day 27

JOYFUL JOINTS

Embark on a journey of gentle movement and tranquility. By focusing on joyfully opening joints, the sequence invites a sense of release and relaxation. The flow benefits various muscle groups, contributing to overall body harmony.

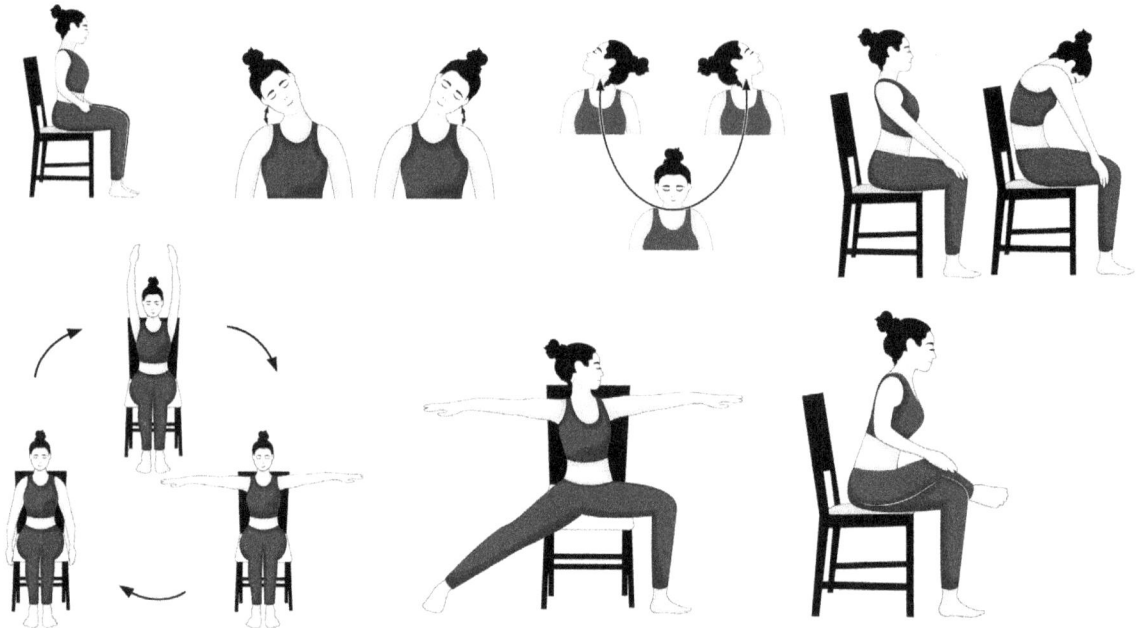

Find a comfortable seated position in the center of the chair, leaving some space between the back of the chair and your back. Rock back and forth until you locate your sit bones. Keep your feet hip-distance apart and flat on the floor. If you prefer, bring your knees together. Take a few deep breaths to center yourself and bring your awareness to the present moment. Begin by gently closing your eyes or softening your gaze. Let go of any distractions and allow your mind to settle. Bring your attention to your breath. Feel the rise and fall of your abdomen with each inhale and exhale. Notice how it feels as it flows in and out of your nose. Follow the breath with your attention, noticing the coolness of the inhale and the warmth of the exhale. Stay for ten breaths, and when ready, move on to the next exercise.

Chair Neck Rolls

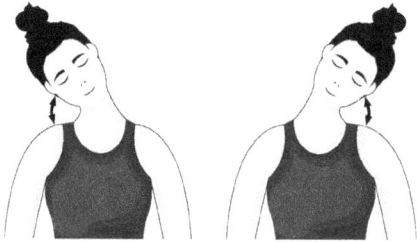

Take a couple of deep breaths. Inhale, move your ear toward the right shoulder, and exhale. Make sure that the neck is long, and the shoulders are relaxed and away from the ears. On the inhale, come back to the center, exhale, and pause before switching sides. Repeat on another side, five times on both sides.

Neck U Rotation Close-Up

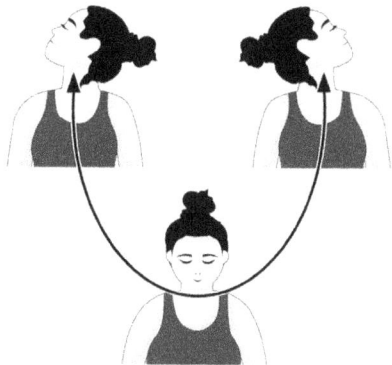

While the movement may seem simple, the improved range of motion helps with other poses and day-to-day activities. Sit comfortably in the chair with a straight spine and feet on the floor. Let your arms rest at your sides. As you inhale, turn your head to the left, exhale, and tuck your chin toward your chest. Inhaling once more, move your chin toward the right shoulder, and exhale, rolling it back to your chest. Alternate between both sides until you return to a neutral position with the chin parallel to the floor. Stay here for two rounds.

Chair Cat-Cow Pose

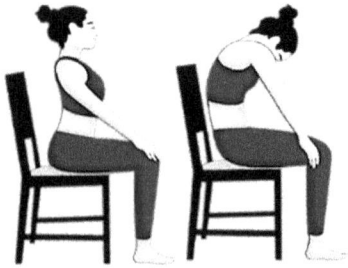

Place your arms on your knees. As you inhale, expand your chest, allowing your head and chin to tilt slightly back. On the exhale, round your spine by curling your chest inward. Ensure your shoulders are relaxed and be aware of the space between your shoulders and earlobes. Practice coordinating your breath with the movement, moving at a comfortable pace. Repeat five to eight times.

Chair Mountain Pose Sweeping Arms Flow

Sit in a mountain pose. Inhale, reaching the arms up, palms facing each other above your head. Exhale and slowly release them down, palms facing down. Inhale, reaching the arms up; exhale with palms facing down. Repeat the sequence for another five times.

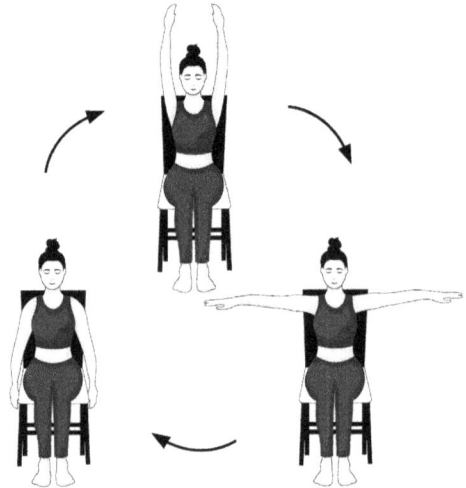

Warrior Pose II Chair

Sit on the edge of the chair. Inhale, and separate the feet. Starting on the left first, open the left leg like a goddess pose, but the left leg only. The knee aligns with the ankle and hip, forming a 90-degree angle. The foot is flat and relaxed, with the toes pointing to the left. Exhale and extend the right leg behind to make it straight in the knee. The right foot is flat here, and the toes point to the front. Make your back straight with your hands resting on the knees. Sit nice and tall. Once the body is comfortable, inhale and extend your arms at shoulder level to a nice T. Ensure the palms are face down and elbows are not bent. Finally, turn your head and gaze at your left fingers. Don't collapse; the torso is straight, and the shoulders are lowered. While here, check the alignment of the legs—the front knee doesn't drop to the side. Stay balanced in the pose. Breathe slowly, deeply, and softly.

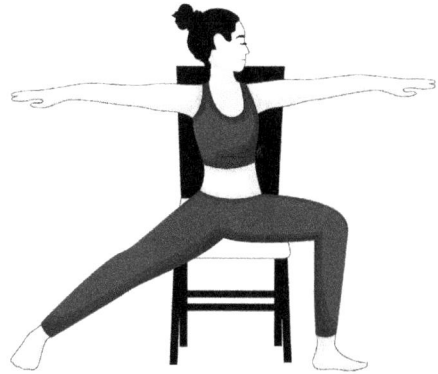

To release the pose: Turn your head back to the center on the exhale. Lower your hands, and realign your legs to the mountain pose. Stay here for a while. Following the previous steps, counter the stretch on the other side.

Chair Pigeon Pose

Sit nice and tall, with your back straight. Now, take a deep breath in as you lift your right leg, holding it gently with your hands, and position it over your left thigh, finding a comfortable sitting position. This seated chair pigeon pose serves to enhance the flexibility and fitness of your hip joint and knee through controlled movement. Once settled into the pose, aim to maintain an erect posture, and take three deep breaths or as many as you require to feel at ease. If you encounter difficulty in crossing one leg over the other, alternatively, lift your right leg, cradling it in your arms for a few seconds before gradually releasing it. Repeat this sequence on the opposite side. Repeat it twice on each side.

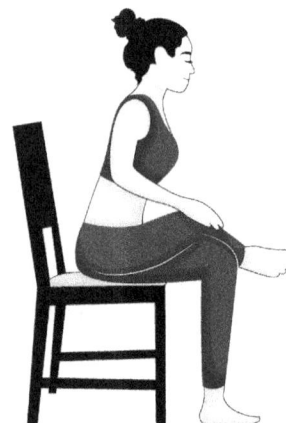

Pause for a moment and tune into your inner sensations. Observe the gentle shifts in your body, the calming of your thoughts, and the emergence of a serene inner peace courtesy of chair yoga. Embrace this opportunity to relax, release, and savor the tranquility within you. It's your time to unwind and bask in the stillness.

CORE STRENGTHENING AND LOWER BODY CARE

As you reach Day 28, the final day of the yoga series, I hope you've already noticed your incredible progress.

Your flexibility has likely increased, your mobility has improved, and you're generally feeling physically and mentally better. Congratulations on completing this journey to a healthier and happier you!

Today's practice is dedicated to strengthening your core and caring for your lower body. Engage in poses focusing on abs, lower back, knees, pelvis, and quadriceps. With each movement, visualize your core gaining strength and your lower body finding comfort.

Embrace this opportunity to nurture these essential muscle groups, fostering a harmonious connection between body and mind.

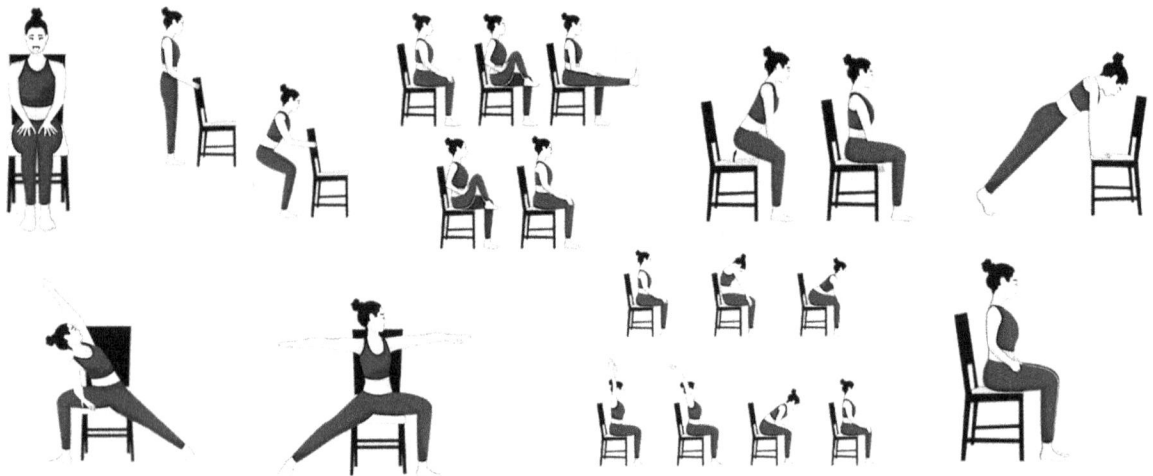

Lions's Breath

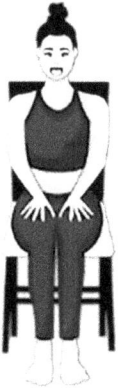

Sit comfortably on the chair and maintain a straight spine. You can lean on your chair backrest—as long as you sit tall with your shoulders lowered. Unbend your arms and stretch out your fingers. This is to imitate a lion's claws. Inhale through the nostrils, then exhale with a loud "ha" from the mouth, extending your tongue as close to the chin as you can. While breathing out, focus on the middle of your forehead or the end of your nose. Fill up with breath, and go back to neutral facial expression. Repeat four to six times.

Let's begin in a mountain pose with your arms pressed against your chest. Take a few deep breaths, and become aware of your surroundings. Breathe in, identify the smell, listen carefully, and identify what you can hear around you. Now, shift your focus to your body. Start from your toes, and slowly scan your way up, paying attention to any sensations, tensions, or areas of tightness that you may feel. Take a few moments to breathe into those areas, and release any tension or discomfort. When ready—move on to the next step.

Mountain Pose Chair to Chair Pose Flow

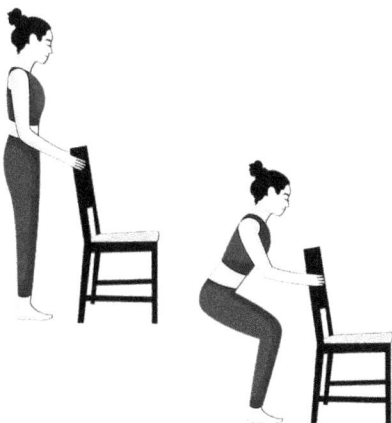

Stand at the back of the chair, holding onto the sides of the chair if help with balance is needed. Inhale, stand tall, grounding down into the soles of the feet, extending the spine upward. Exhale and sit weight back into heels. If you need a bigger challenge—your toes can be lifted to exaggerate the weight in the heels. Lower belly pulled in. The

28 Days of Chair Yoga for Seniors

knees should be positioned behind the toes. Keep length in the spine and the back of the neck. Hold for three breaths. Repeat twice.

Seated Low Lunge Pose

This easy flow will help stretch your feet, ankles, hips, and knees and strengthen your pelvic floor. Sit tall with both feet on the floor and sit bones grounded on the chair. Inhale, and bend your right knee toward your chest.

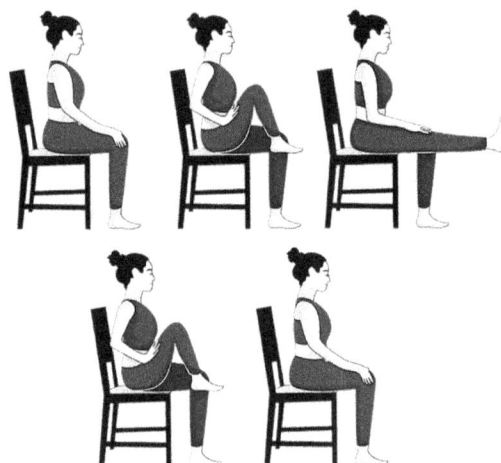

Exhale, and extend your leg out. Toes up toward the ceiling. Inhale, and bring it back by bending your right knee toward your chest. Exhale, and place your foot on the floor. Repeat on the other side—a total of five times for each leg. If you need to bend your knee toward your chest, you can grab under the knee and support your move.

Easy Pose Chair to Chair Pose Flow

Sit tall, feet flat on the floor, hands on your lap. Inhale and lean forward, activating the glutes and quads. Lift hips, knees slightly bent. Look ahead, hands on knees. Exhale, lower to the seat. Repeat five times.

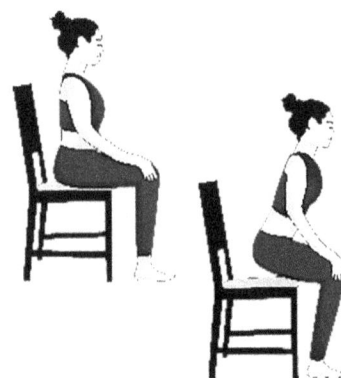

166

Plank Pose with Chair

Place your hands on the seat of the chair. Stack shoulders over hands, walk your feet back, hip-distance apart. Depending on your body's abilities, walk your feet as far as you feel comfortable. You can be on your toes or feet flat, core engaged. Observe your shoulders being stacked over your wrists. Keep your spine straight. Long line from shoulders to feet. Hold five long, deep breaths or less.

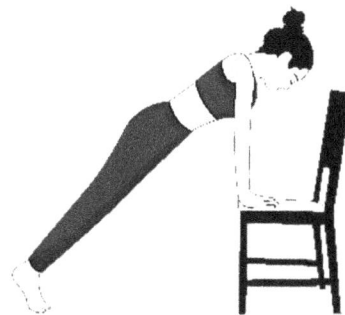

Extended Side Angle Pose Variation Elbow Arm Chair

Inhale, turn your right foot outward and place the right thigh on the chair.

Exhale, extend your left leg to the left side of the chair while lifting your right arm and stretching the side as you gaze upward.

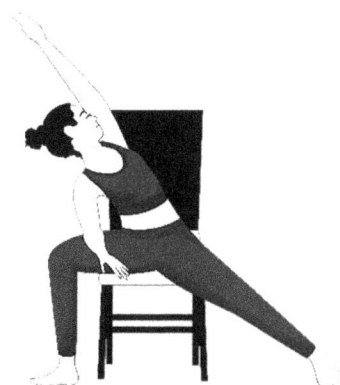

Hold the pose for three breaths, inhaling and exhaling deeply. Repeat on the other side.

Warrior Pose II Chair

Sit on the edge of the chair. Inhale, and separate the feet. Starting on the left first, open the left leg like a goddess pose, but the left leg only. The knee aligns with the ankle and hip, forming a 90-degree angle.

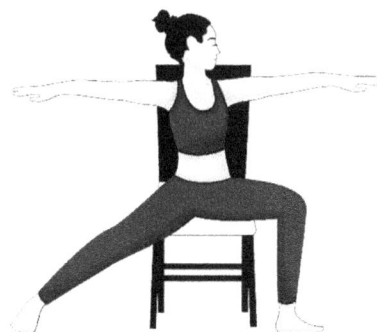

The foot is flat and relaxed, with the toes pointing to the left. Exhale and extend the right leg behind to make it straight in the knee. The right foot is flat here, and the toes point to the front.

Make your back straight with your hands resting on the knees. Sit nice and tall. Once the body is comfortable, inhale and extend your arms at shoulder level to a nice T.

Ensure the palms are face down and elbows are not bent.

Finally, turn your head and gaze at your left fingers. Don't collapse; the torso is straight, and the shoulders are lowered.

While here, check the alignment of the legs—the front knee doesn't drop to the side. Stay balanced in the pose. Breathe slowly, deeply, and softly.

To release the pose:

- Turn your head back to the center on the exhale.
- Lower your hands and realign your legs to the mountain pose.
- Stay here for a while.
- Following the previous steps, counter the stretch on the other side.

Seated Half Forward Fold Pose Chair Flow

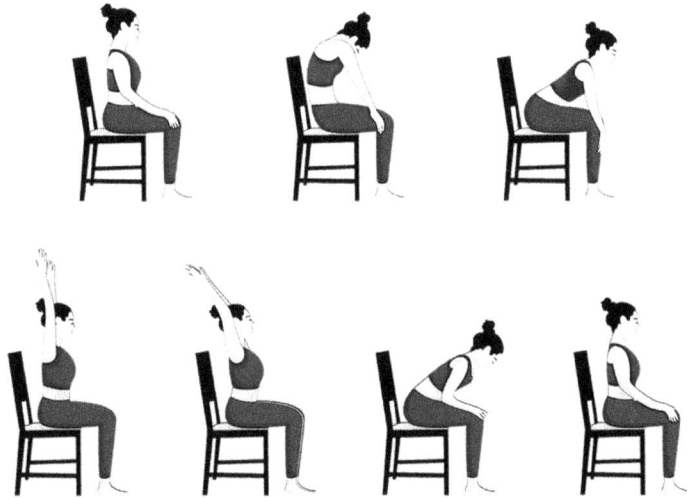

Sit comfortably in a chair, spine tall, and feel grounded on the floor. On the inhale, round your spine, and on the exhale, lean forward. Allow your hands to hold onto your knees, and lean back, arching your back. Inhale, and raise your arms above your head. And if you feel comfortable, slightly lean back. On the exhale, fold over your thighs. Come back to the neutral position. Repeat the sequence. Work with a breath.

Before you move on to other things, savor the good you've done during this session. Feel the support of the chair beneath you, grounding you in the present moment. Close your eyes gently, keep a soft gaze, and focus inward. Be aware of the rhythm of your breath. Notice how gently your chest and abdomen rise and fall with each inhale and exhale. Allow any remaining tension or stress to melt away with every breath out, leaving you in a state of profound relaxation. Imagine a sense of calm washing over you, like a gentle wave lapping at the shore. Take a moment to express gratitude for your dedicated time to yourself and your well-being. Recognize the peace that resides within you, always accessible through the practice of chair yoga. Now, gently open your eyes, carry this newfound sense of serenity, and prepare to transition to the next step with renewed energy and mindfulness.

3 Bonus Sequences

As you have learned, all the routines start with being aware of the present: check if the shoulders are relaxed, keep your spine straight, and guide your attention to your breath. Sit nice and tall in a mountain pose position, feeling the chair supporting your body. Bring your thoughts into the present moment, leaving any distractions or worries behind. Take a few deep, grounding breaths, inhaling positivity and exhaling tension. Once you're ready, proceed with the next exercise.

When you conclude your chair yoga sequence, use one of the breathing techniques you've learned during this 28-day chair yoga journey. You can do alternate nostril breathing, Lion's Breath, or three-part breathing—whichever resonates with you today. These techniques will help you further relax your body and mind. Or you can sit and take a moment to bask in the serenity that your practice has cultivated. Feel your body, scan for any lingering tension, and observe how it may have shifted during your session. Embrace this newfound sense of peace and mindfulness. When you're ready, gently open your eyes, knowing you can carry this tranquility with you as you continue your day.

First: Muscle Activation
Hip Openers, Knees, Pelvic, Quadriceps, Shoulders, and Upper Back

Embrace hip openness for mobility and tension release. Show your knees some gentle care for flexibility. Nourish your pelvic region to enhance core balance. Strengthen and stretch quadriceps for lower body power. Extend flexibility to shoulders and arms, relieving upper body tension. Find upper back relief through mindful stretches.

Each movement enriches your muscles with vitality. This routine harmonizes diverse muscle groups, nurturing both body and mind in perfect unity.

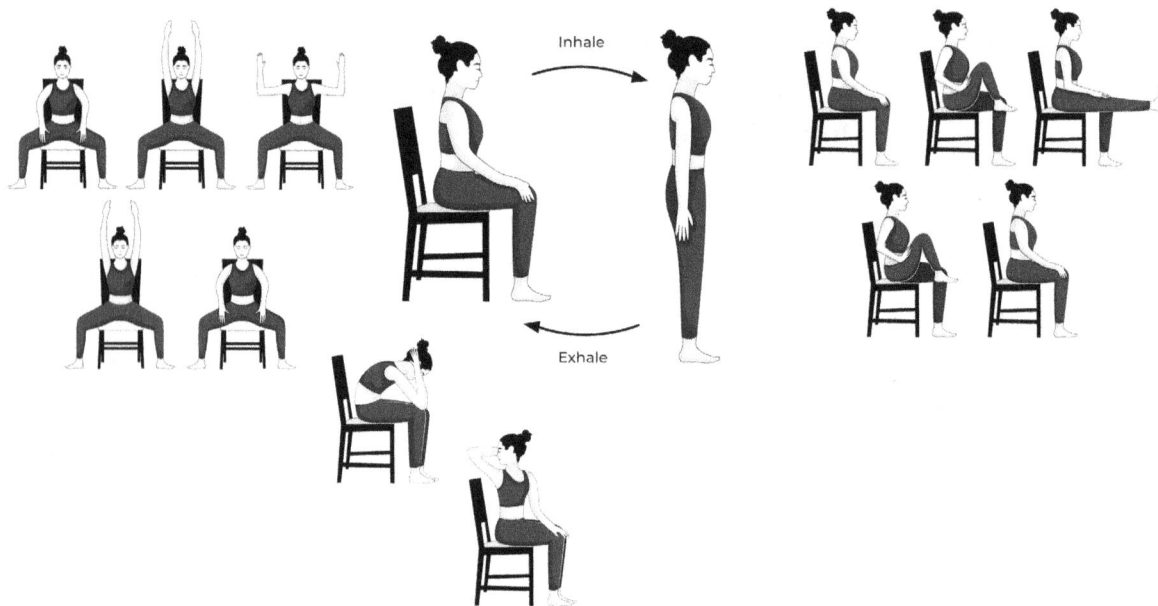

Goddess Pose on Chair Arms Flow

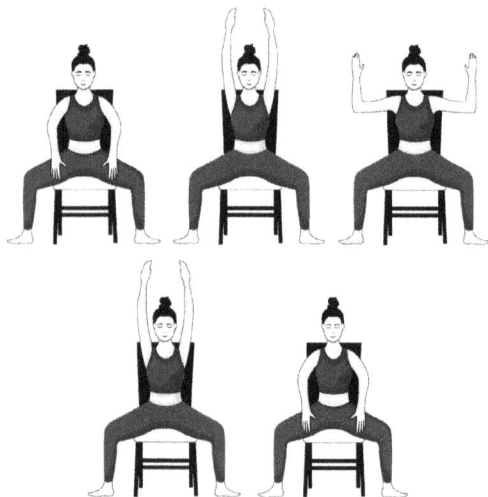

Inhale to rotate the hips outward, bringing the feet to 120 degrees, with toes pointing sideways and knees bent. Gently push out the inner thighs as you plant both feet firmly on the floor. Raise your arms overhead—palms facing each other—keeping shoulders away from ears. Exhale while bending elbows so forearms are perpendicular and palms are facing forward (cactus arms). Hold for thirty seconds before inhaling to extend arms up again with palms together. Lower arms back down at shoulder level in an exhale, and place hands on inner thighs before inhaling again to raise them. Complete four to six repetitions of this flow, coordinating breathing as needed, then release and relax.

Chair Mountain Pose Standing Flow

This is a simple-looking but powerful short sequence to develop strength in the lower body. Engage your thighs and glutes, and on the inhale, stand up and slowly, on the exhale, sit down. Repeat five times. If you need a challenge, slow down when sitting down—feel your quads and hamstrings in action.

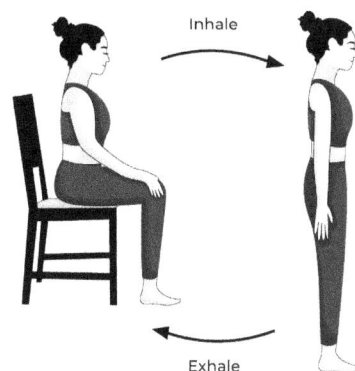

Seated Low Lunge Pose

This easy flow will help stretch your feet, ankles, hips, and knees and strengthen your pelvic floor. Sit tall with both feet on the floor and sit bones grounded on the chair. Inhale, and bend your right knee toward your chest.

Exhale, and extend your leg out. Toes up toward the ceiling. Inhale, and bring it back by bending your right knee toward your chest. Exhale, and place your foot on the floor. Repeat on the other side—a total of five times for each leg. If you need to bend your knee toward your chest, you can grab under the knee and support your move.

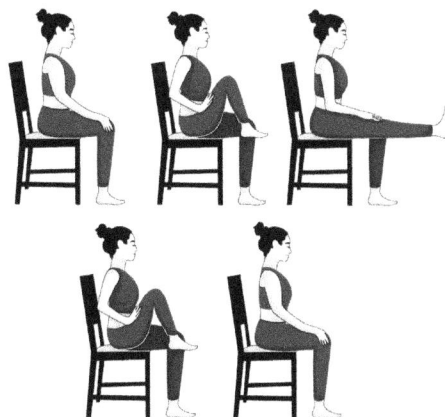

Seated Chair One Hand Behind Head Elbow Knee Flow

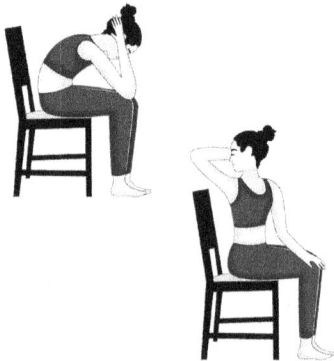

Place your palms with elbows bent at the back of your head. On the exhale, bend forward at the hips, bringing your elbows together, and lean on your knees with your elbows. On the inhale, sit up straight and leave your left arm resting on the thighs. At the same time, bring your right elbow back and look over that elbow. On the exhale, bend forward again, bringing your elbows together.

Inhale—sit up straight once more while bringing your left elbow back and look over that elbow. Repeat this sequence, coordinating your breath with the movements four times.

Second: Balanced Muscle Engagement Abs, Knees, Quadriceps, and Shoulder Arms

Immerse yourself in a chair yoga routine meticulously curated to activate essential muscle groups.

Strengthen your core, cultivating stability and balance. Tenderly nurture knee health with stretches that enhance flexibility. Strengthen and stretch these vital leg muscles for overall lower body well-being. Elevate upper body flexibility and stability, releasing tension.

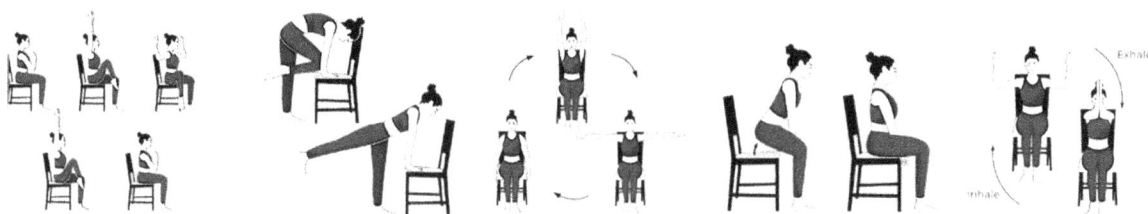

Seated Low Lunge Variation Chair Arms Raised Flow

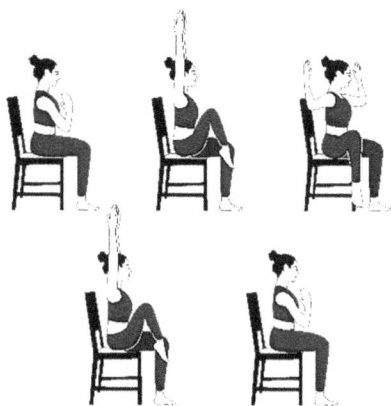

Sit up nice and tall in a mountain position. On the inhale, reach your arms and right knee up together. On the exhale, open your arms to a cactus position—arms bend at the elbows at the shoulder level. Simultaneously, bring your right knee to the side. Inhale, and reach both arms back up toward the sky, lifting your knee toward your chest at a center. Exhale, and put your right knee down, returning your arms to the prayer position. Repeat on the other side. Repeat it twice on each side. If you need a challenge—repeat it three times.

Standing Table Top Pose with Knee to Nose Flow Chair

Begin by standing tall and upright, squarely facing the chair seat. Inhale deeply, allowing the breath to steady you. On the exhale, gently place your hands on the chair, creating a supportive connection, envisioning your neck as an extension of your spine. Continue exhaling as you lengthen your spine and direct the extension through your head. Glide your right leg behind you to its fullest extent. As you exhale, draw the right knee toward your nose, curving it inward. Inhale again, send the leg back by extending it, creating length, and then exhale to bring the knee toward your nose again. Repeat this fluid sequence a total of six times on one side. Return to your stance in the mountain pose, taking a moment to stand firmly and breathe. Mirror the sequence on the opposite side, maintaining your focus and intention throughout.

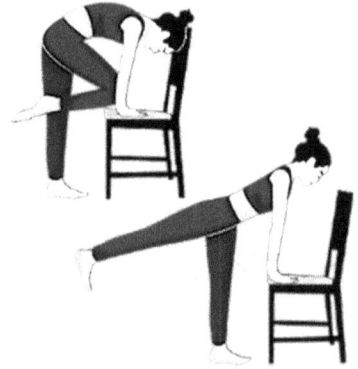

Chair Mountain Pose Sweeping Arms Flow

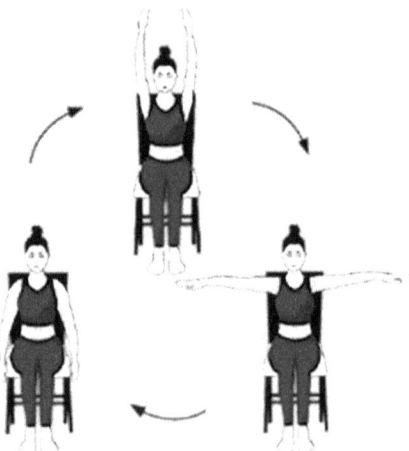

Sit in a mountain pose. Inhale, reaching the arms up, palms facing each other above your head. Exhale and slowly release them down, palms facing down. Inhale, reaching the arms up; exhale with palms facing down. Repeat the sequence for another five times.

Easy Pose Chair to Chair Pose Flow

Sit tall, feet flat on the floor, hands on your lap.

Inhale, lean forward and activate glutes and quads. Lift hips, knees slightly bent. Look ahead, hands on knees. Exhale, lower to the seat. Repeat five times.

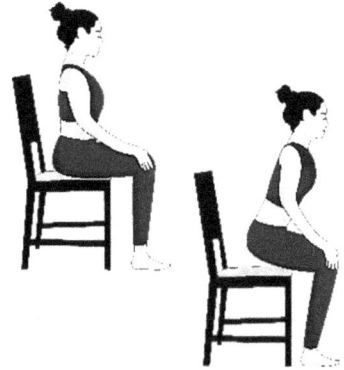

Seated Cactus Arms Flow Chair

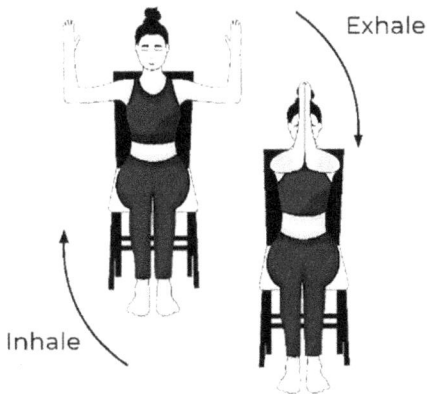

Cactus arms, elbows in line with shoulders, wrists stacked over elbows. Spread the fingers and point them up. Breathe in, and bring your arms to the side with your elbows bent as pictured. Take a deep breath, lift through the chest, and squeeze the shoulder blades together. Listen to your body. As you exhale, bring your elbows, forearms, and hands together. Inhale, open your arms into a cactus position, and squeeze your shoulder blades together. Repeat the flow three to five times. Work on coordinating the flow with the breath.

Third: Revitalizing Foundation Feet and Ankles, Hip Openers

Embark on a chair yoga routine that rejuvenates your body's foundation and promotes fluid movement. Embrace stretches that provide comfort and support to these essential areas. Cultivate fluidity and ease in your hip joints, enhancing overall mobility.

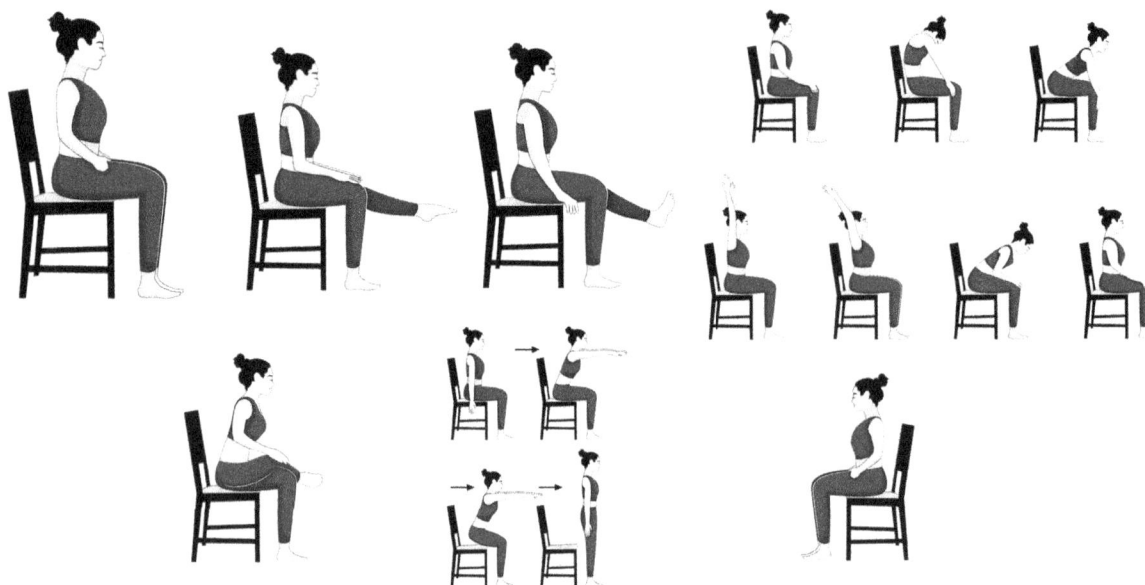

Chair Flexing Foot Pose

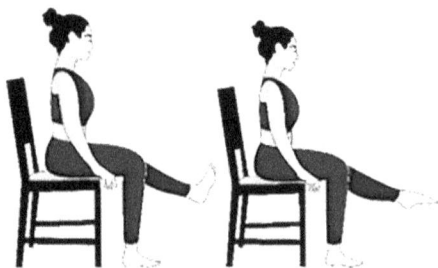

Lift your right leg, and point the toes away from you. As you inhale, lift your toes toward your face and press the heel away. Exhale, and point your toes outward. Repeat this sequence five times before switching to the other leg.

Seated Half Forward Fold Pose Chair Flow

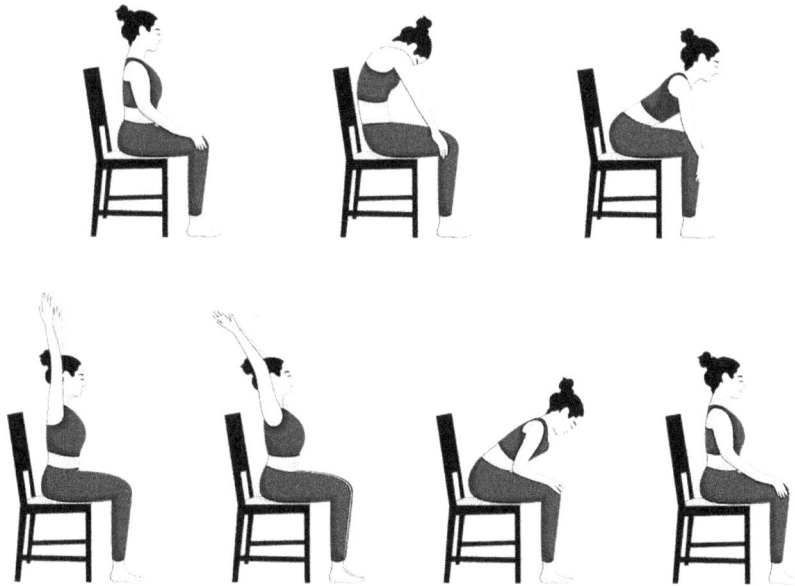

Sit comfortably in a chair, spine tall, and feel grounded on the floor. On the inhale, round your spine, and on the exhale, lean forward. Allow your hands to hold onto your knees, and lean back, arching your back. Inhale, and raise your arms above your head. And if you feel comfortable, slightly lean back. On the exhale, fold over your thighs. Come back to the neutral position. Repeat the sequence. Work with a breath.

Chair Pigeon Pose

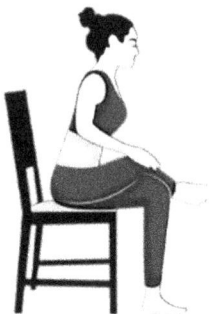

Sit nice and tall, with your back straight. Now, take a deep breath in as you lift your right leg, holding it gently with your hands, and position it over your left thigh, finding a comfortable sitting position. This seated chair pigeon pose serves to enhance the flexibility and fitness of your hip joint and knee through controlled movement. Once settled into the pose, aim to maintain an erect posture, and take three deep breaths or as many as you require to feel at ease. If you encounter difficulty in crossing one leg over the other, alternatively, lift your right leg, cradling it in your arms for a few seconds before gradually releasing it. Repeat this sequence on the opposite side. Repeat it twice on each side.

Chair Mountain Pose Stand-Up Flow

Start in a mountain pose. The spine is nice and tall, shoulders rolled back. Reach your arms forward to help you lift your hips off the chair. Hold this position for a couple of breaths; if not, stand up. Feel the ground under your feet. Sit back down with your arms next to you. Repeat five more times.

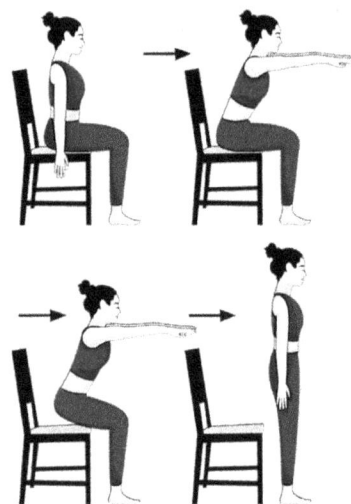

Conclusion

Like anything, yoga takes time and practice to get from good to incredible, and your body is different from everyone else. Use your intuition; stop if it hurts.

Attempting any exercise too extreme (the definition of which changes with age, regardless of fitness) or beyond your fitness level makes injury more likely. This is as true with yoga as any other form of exercise. This is why I actively encourage you—if in doubt —to consult your doctor. If there is any pain—stop it. Don't push if you feel that your body cannot do it.

Chair yoga is more than modified poses. It is about self-awareness. It is about self-acceptance and honesty. When you take those elements out and make it a "sport," with competition, ego, and pushing yourself to the edge as goals, you are likely to hurt yourself.

Each person must find the limit between helping and hurting their own body.

So, whether you follow this program diligently or adapt it to your needs, always remember your "why." Stay consistent, embrace your journey, and respect your body's limits.

As you leave the pages of this guide and continue your chair yoga practice, know that you can transform your life—one gentle pose, one deep breath, and one day at a time. Embrace the benefits of chair yoga, and may it bring you a renewed sense of vitality, strength, and inner peace. Your journey has just begun, and the path ahead has endless possibilities. Chair yoga is your companion on this voyage, guiding you toward a healthier, happier, and more balanced life.

And the last thing before you go: Simply by sharing your honest opinion of this book on Amazon, you'll show other readers that they can benefit too—and exactly where they can find the guidance they need to make sure they do.

Thank you for being so supportive. With your help, I can make sure that the message reaches even more people.

You Could Be Key to Someone Else's Yoga Journey

TAKE A MOMENT TO SHARE YOUR THOUGHTS!

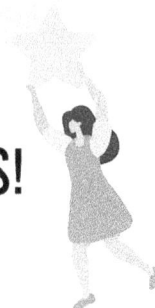

Thank you so much for your support. No matter what might hold us back from standing yoga, we can still access its astounding potential ... And with your help, I can make sure that the message reaches even more people.

Appendix

Day 1: Neck, Shoulder, Arms, and Upper Back Relief

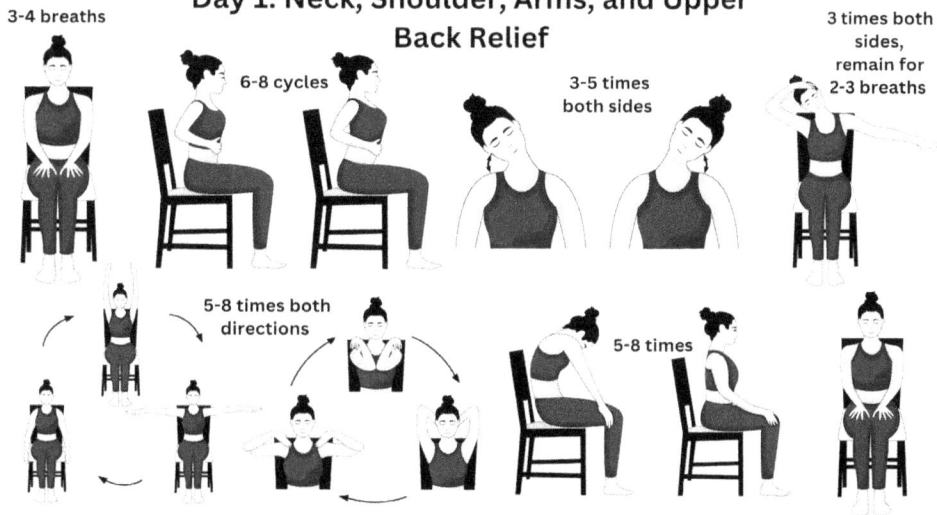

3-4 breaths

6-8 cycles

3-5 times both sides

3 times both sides, remain for 2-3 breaths

5-8 times both directions

5-8 times

Day 2: Glutes, Lower Back, and Knees Strengthening

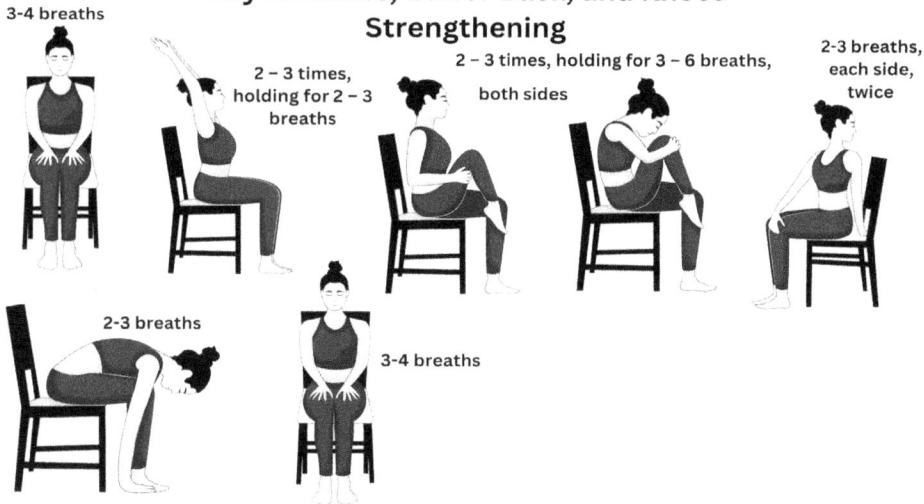

3-4 breaths

2 – 3 times, holding for 2 – 3 breaths

2 – 3 times, holding for 3 – 6 breaths, both sides

2-3 breaths, each side, twice

2-3 breaths

3-4 breaths

Day 3: Feet, Ankles, Hamstrings, and Quadriceps Care

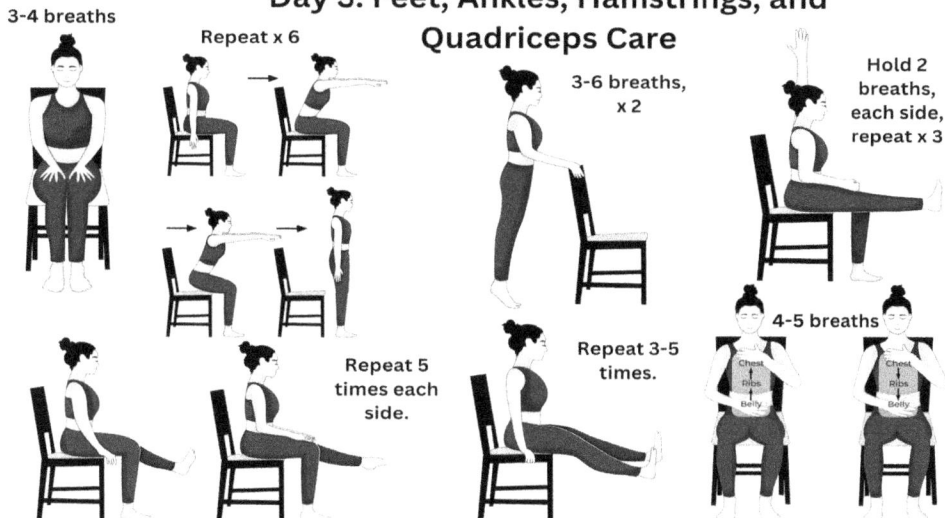

3-4 breaths

Repeat x 6

3-6 breaths, x 2

Hold 2 breaths, each side, repeat x 3

Repeat 5 times each side.

Repeat 3-5 times.

4-5 breaths

Chest
Ribs
Belly

Chest
Ribs
Belly

Day 4: Shoulder and Arms Mobility

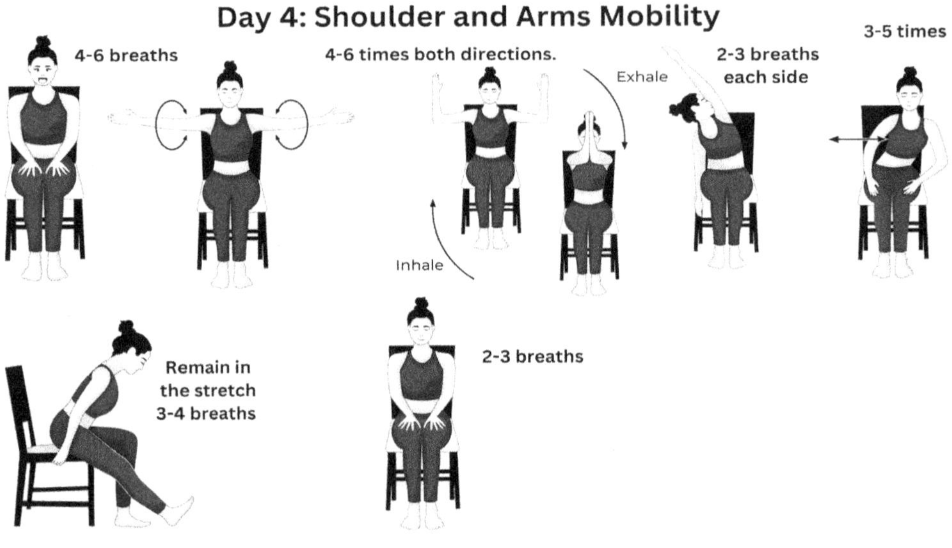

4-6 breaths

4-6 times both directions.

Exhale

2-3 breaths each side

3-5 times

Inhale

Remain in the stretch 3-4 breaths

2-3 breaths

Day 5: Hip Openers, Knees, Upper Back, and Pelvic Release

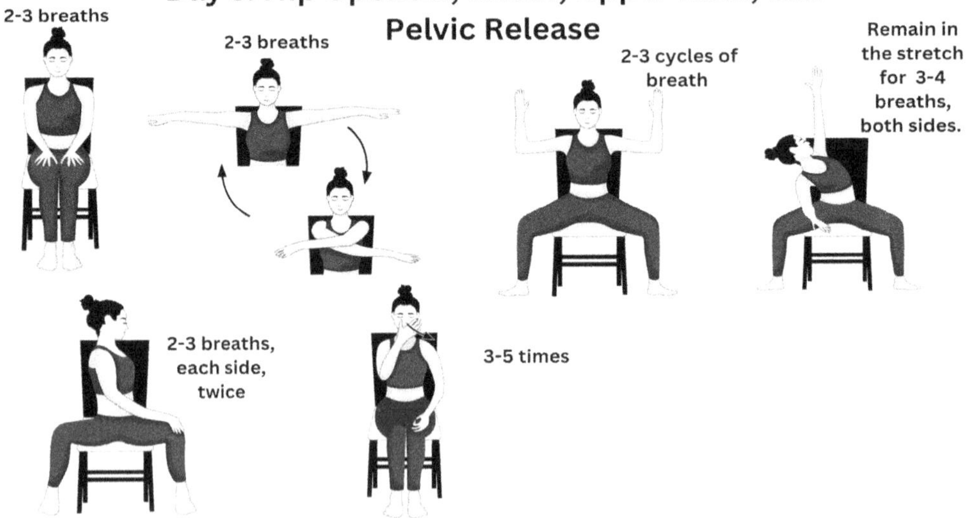

2-3 breaths

2-3 breaths

2-3 cycles of breath

Remain in the stretch for 3-4 breaths, both sides.

2-3 breaths, each side, twice

3-5 times

Day 6: Shoulder, Arms, and Wrist Exercises

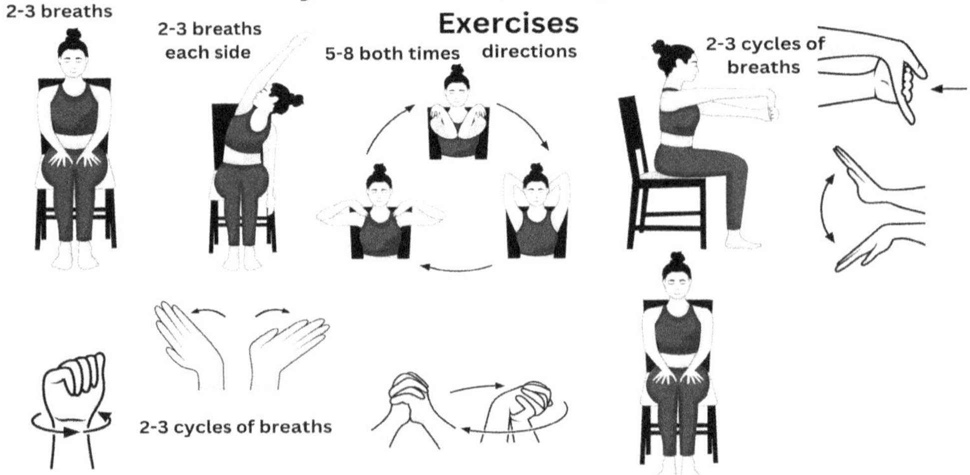

2-3 breaths

2-3 breaths each side

5-8 both times   directions

2-3 cycles of breaths

2-3 cycles of breaths

Day 7: Lower Back, Hamstrings, and Neck Relaxation

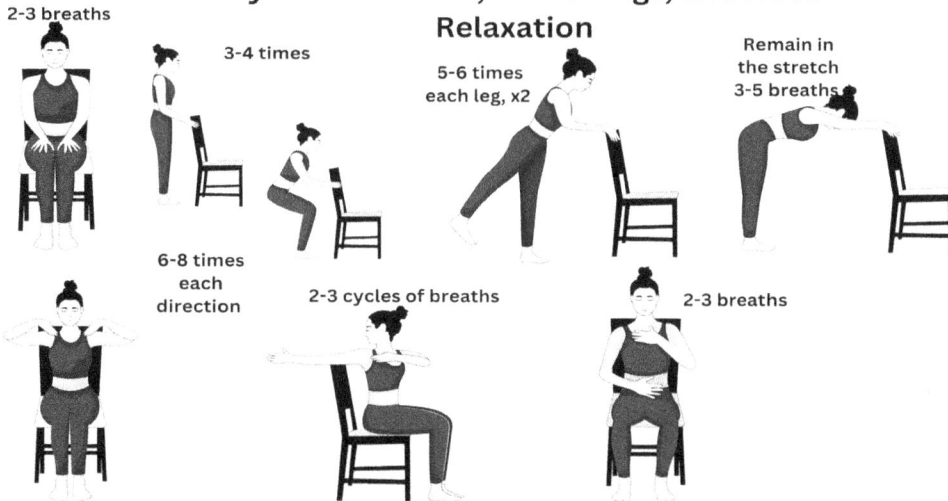

2-3 breaths

3-4 times

5-6 times each leg, x2

Remain in the stretch 3-5 breaths

6-8 times each direction

2-3 cycles of breaths

2-3 breaths

Day 8: Hamstrings, Hip Openers, Quadriceps, and Upper Back Flow

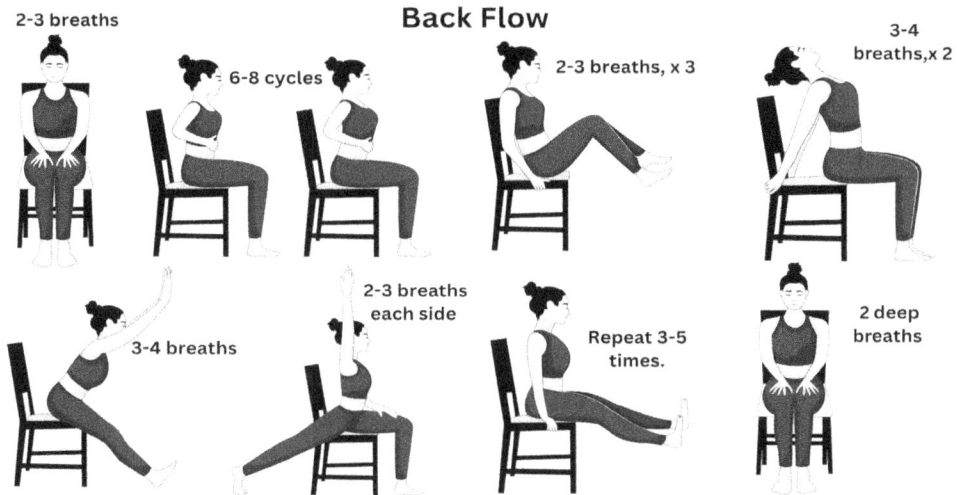

2-3 breaths

6-8 cycles

2-3 breaths, x 3

3-4 breaths, x 2

3-4 breaths

2-3 breaths each side

Repeat 3-5 times.

2 deep breaths

Day 9: Empowering Lower Back, Neck, Shoulders, Arms, and Upper Back

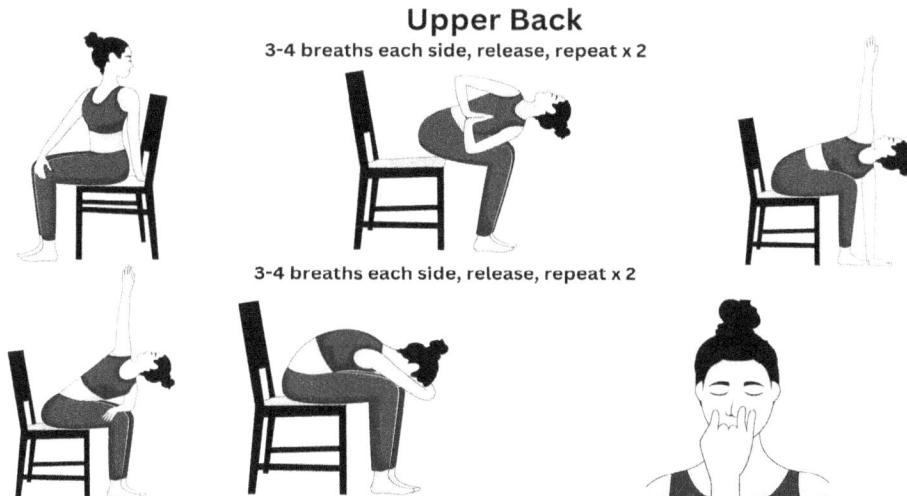

3-4 breaths each side, release, repeat x 2

3-4 breaths each side, release, repeat x 2

Day 10: Abdominals, Hip Openers, Knees, Quadriceps, and Upper Back Revitalization

2 deep breaths

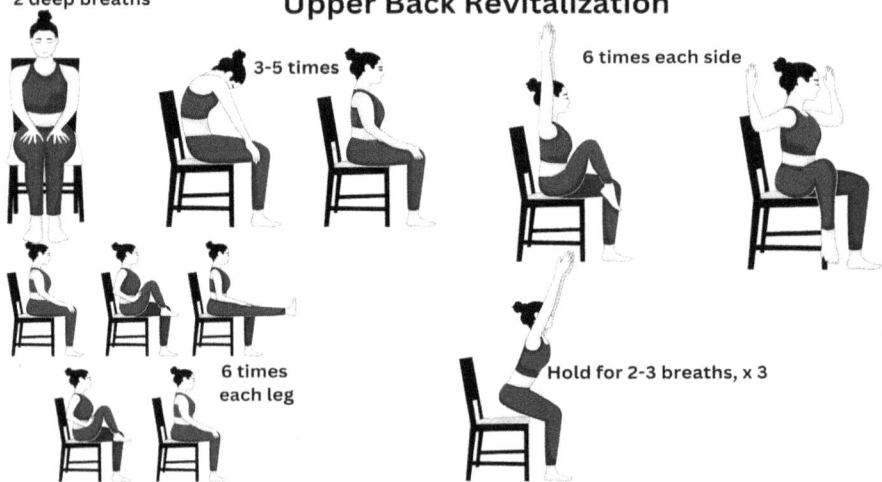

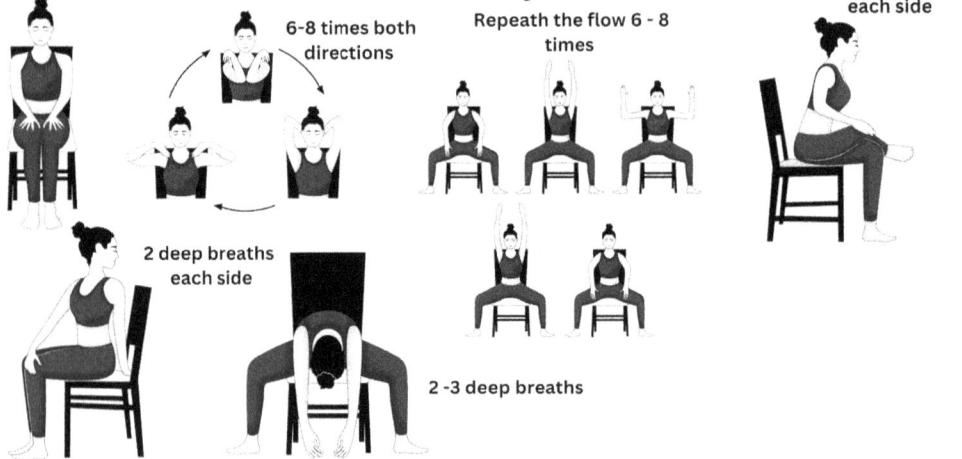

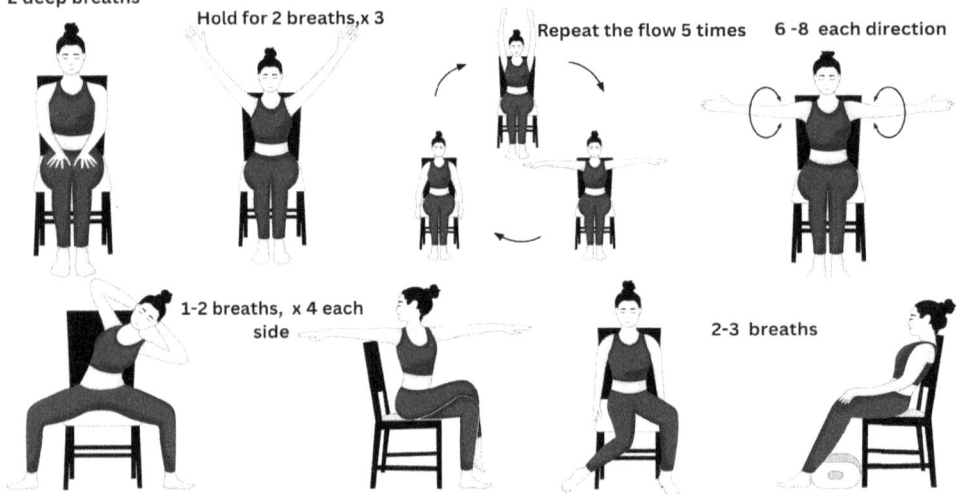

3-5 times

6 times each side

6 times each leg

Hold for 2-3 breaths, x 3

Day 11: Upper Back, Hip, Pelvic, Shoulder, and Arm Harmony

2 deep breaths

6-8 times both directions

Repeath the flow 6 - 8 times

2 deep breaths each side

2 deep breaths each side

2 -3 deep breaths

Day 12: Psoas Release for Upper Back Comfort

2 deep breaths

Hold for 2 breaths, x 3

Repeat the flow 5 times

6 -8 each direction

1-2 breaths, x 4 each side

2-3 breaths

Day 13: Abdominals, Feet and Ankles, Hips, and Lower Back Wellness

2 deep breaths

3-4 times

3-4 times

3-4 times each side

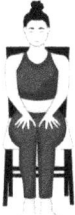 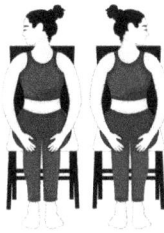 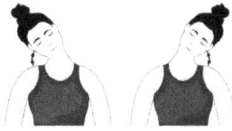 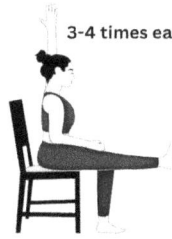

3-4 breaths, each side

2-3 breaths

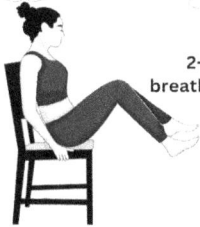 2-3 breaths, x 3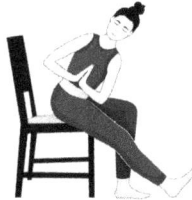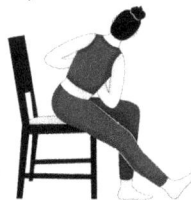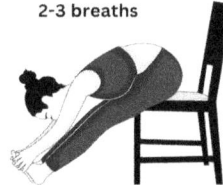

Day 14: Hip Openers, Lower Back, and Neck Relief with Core Activation

3-5 breathing cycles

3-5 times

3-4 breaths, each side

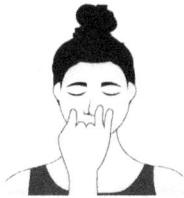 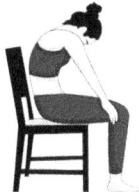 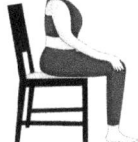 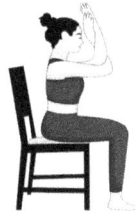 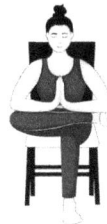

3-4 breaths

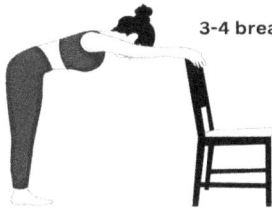 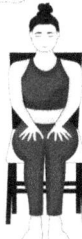 3-4 breaths

Day 15: Hamstrings, Hips, Knees, and Quadriceps Care

Remain in the pose for 3-4 breaths on each side for each exercise

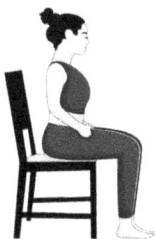 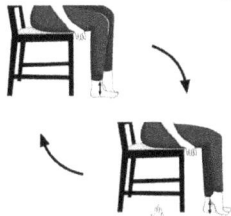 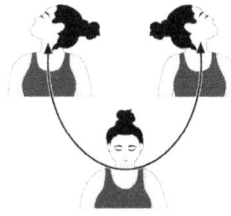 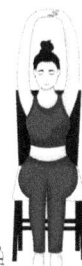

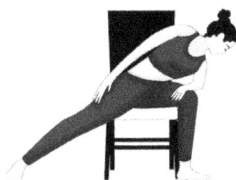 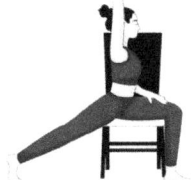 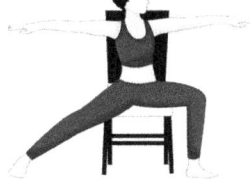 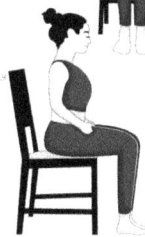

Day 16: Feet and Ankles Renewal – Completing a Balanced Journey

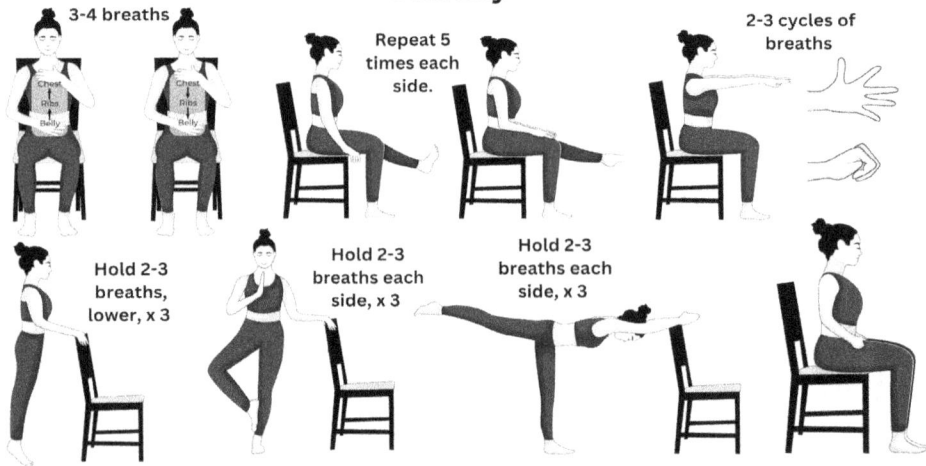

3-4 breaths

Chest
Ribs
Belly

Chest
Ribs
Belly

Repeat 5 times each side.

2-3 cycles of breaths

Hold 2-3 breaths, lower, x 3

Hold 2-3 breaths each side, x 3

Hold 2-3 breaths each side, x 3

Day 17: Holistic Balance – A Full Body Journey

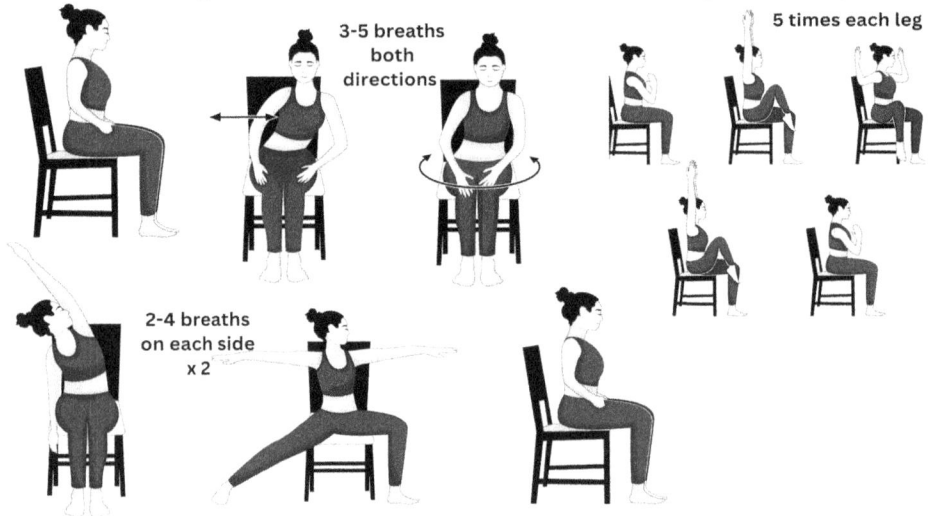

3-5 breaths both directions

5 times each leg

2-4 breaths on each side x 2

Day 18: Nurturing Feet, Ankles, Hip Openers, and Quadriceps

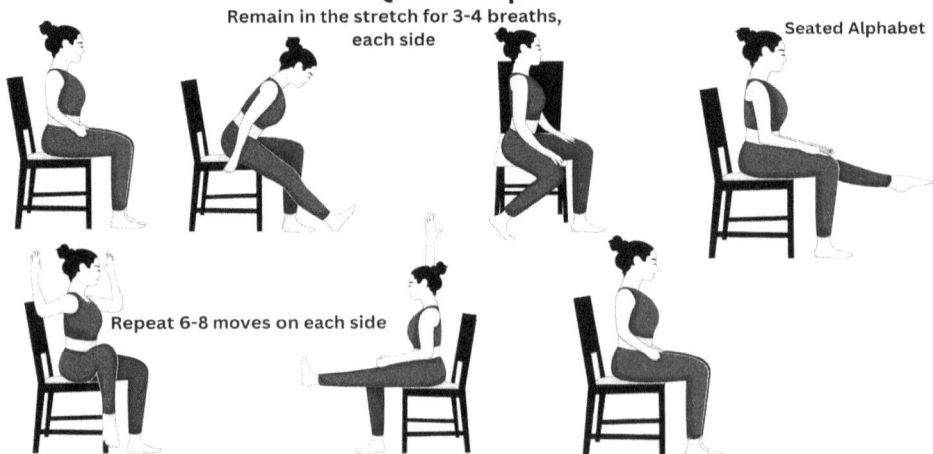

Remain in the stretch for 3-4 breaths, each side

Seated Alphabet

Repeat 6-8 moves on each side

Day 19: Biceps Triceps, Abs, and Knees

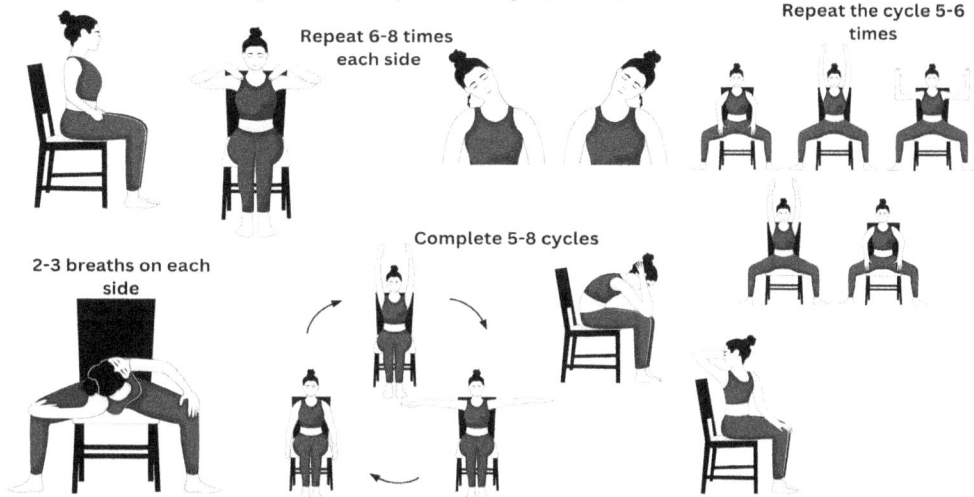

Repeat 6-8 times each side

Repeat the cycle 5-6 times

Complete 5-8 cycles

2-3 breaths on each side

Day 20: Hip Openers, Psoas Muscle, Hamstrings, Abs, and Lower Back Harmony

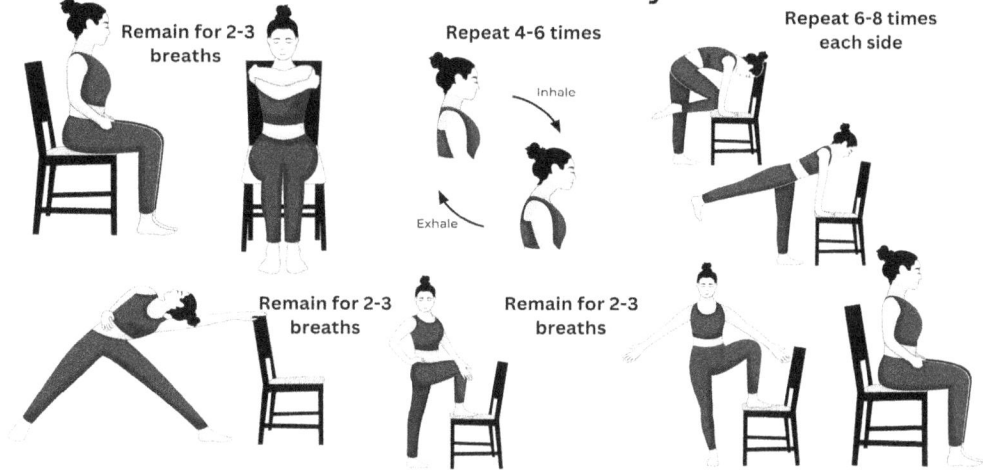

Remain for 2-3 breaths

Repeat 4-6 times

Inhale

Exhale

Repeat 6-8 times each side

Remain for 2-3 breaths

Remain for 2-3 breaths

Day 21: Gentle Restoration – Neck, Biceps, Hips, and Knees

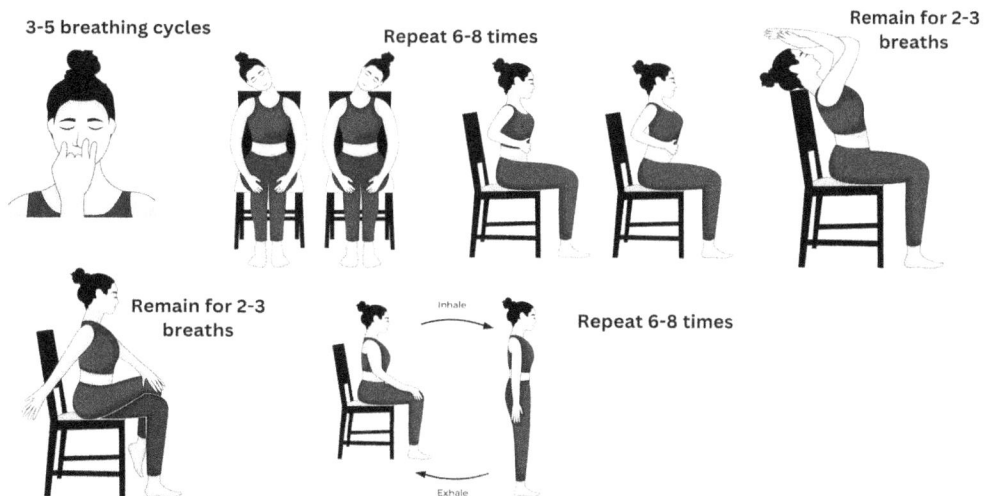

3-5 breathing cycles

Repeat 6-8 times

Remain for 2-3 breaths

Remain for 2-3 breaths

Inhale

Exhale

Repeat 6-8 times

191

Day 22: Hamstrings, Abs, Knees, Shoulders, and Gluteus Strength

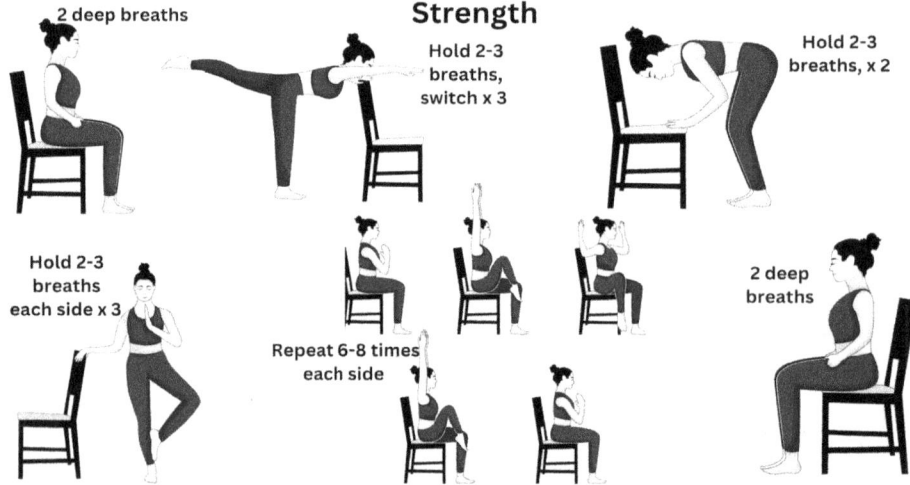

2 deep breaths

Hold 2-3 breaths, switch x 3

Hold 2-3 breaths, x 2

Hold 2-3 breaths each side x 3

Repeat 6-8 times each side

2 deep breaths

Day 23: Comprehensive Renewal Routine

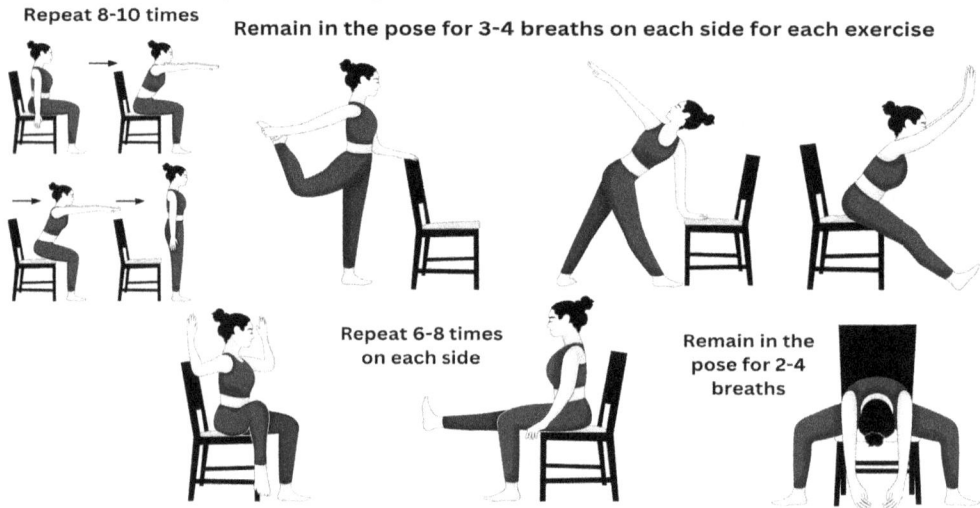

Repeat 8-10 times

Remain in the pose for 3-4 breaths on each side for each exercise

Repeat 6-8 times on each side

Remain in the pose for 2-4 breaths

Day 24: Comprehensive Muscle Focus

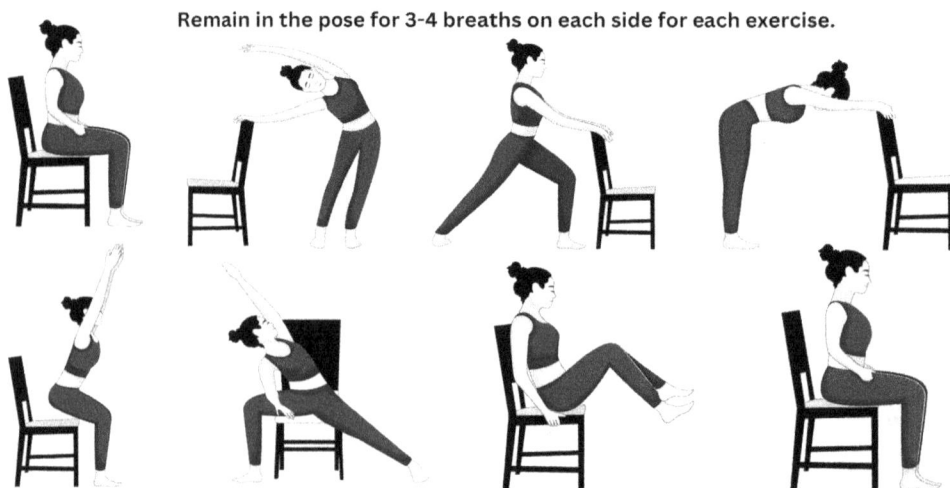

Remain in the pose for 3-4 breaths on each side for each exercise.

Day 25: Muscle Activation

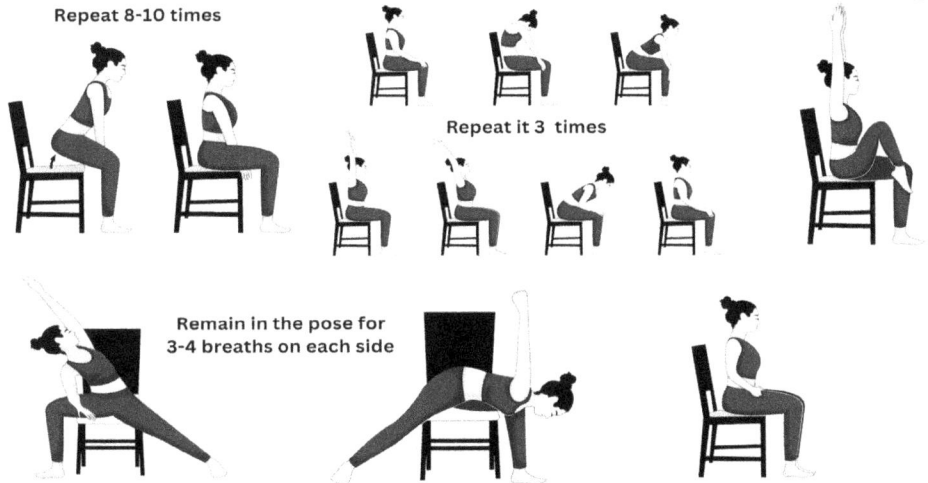

Repeat 8-10 times

6-8 times each leg

Repeat it 3 times

Remain in the pose for
3-4 breaths on each side

Day 26: Sun Salutation on the Chair

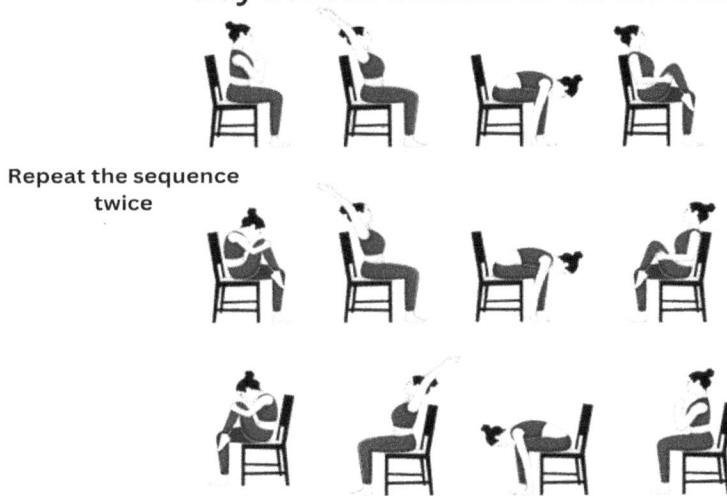

Repeat the sequence
twice

Day 27: Joyful Joints

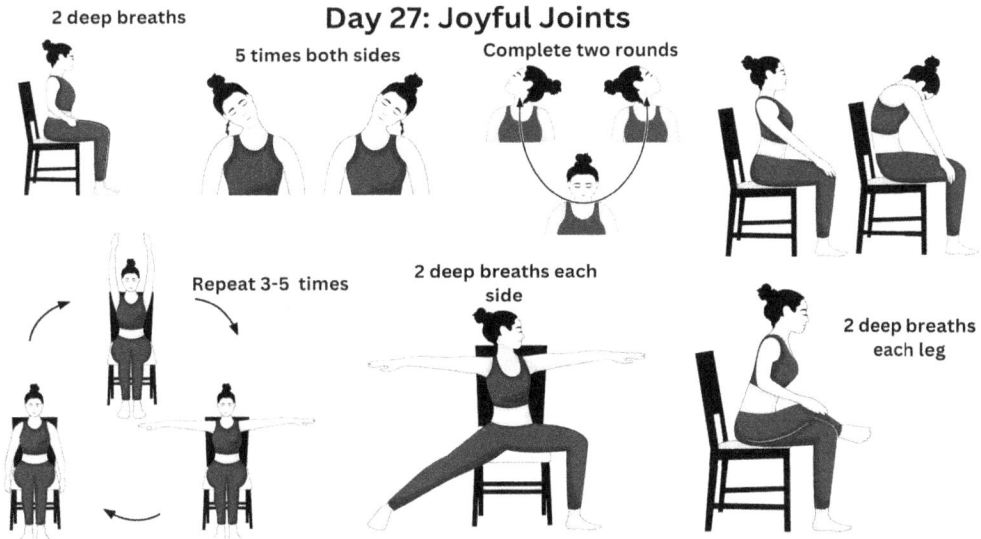

2 deep breaths

5 times both sides

Complete two rounds

Repeat 3-5 times

2 deep breaths each
side

2 deep breaths
each leg

Day 28: Core Strengthening and Lower Body Care

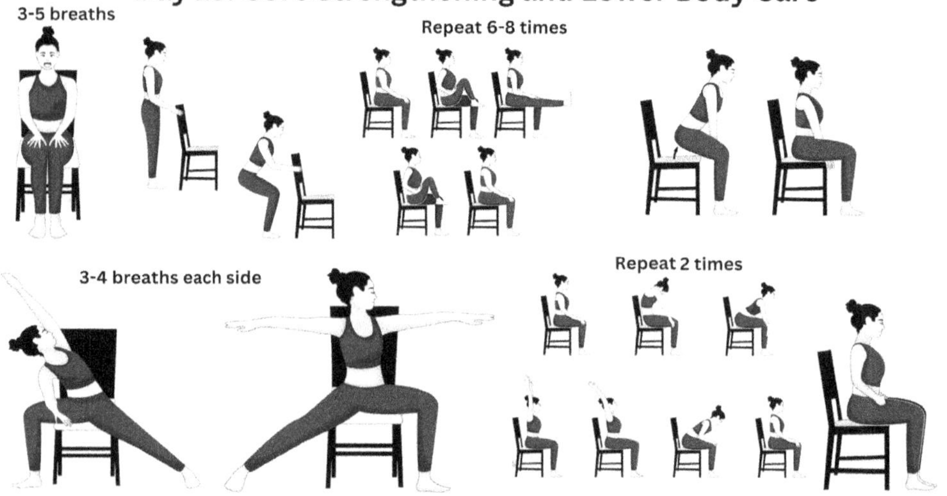

3-5 breaths

Repeat 6-8 times

3-4 breaths each side

Repeat 2 times

Bonus Sequence

First: Muscle Activation – Hip Openers, Knees, Pelvic, Quadriceps, Shoulders, and Upper Back

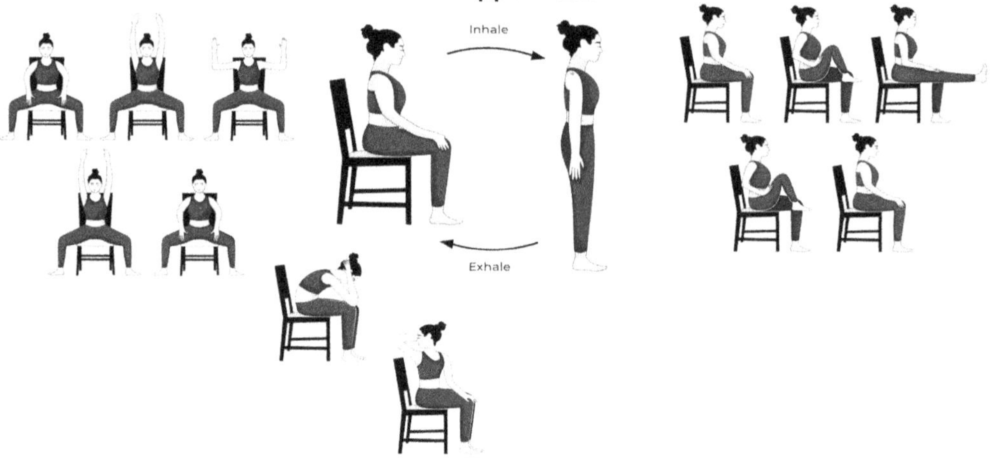

Inhale

Exhale

Second: Balanced Muscle Engagement – Abs, Knees, Quadriceps, and Shoulder Arms

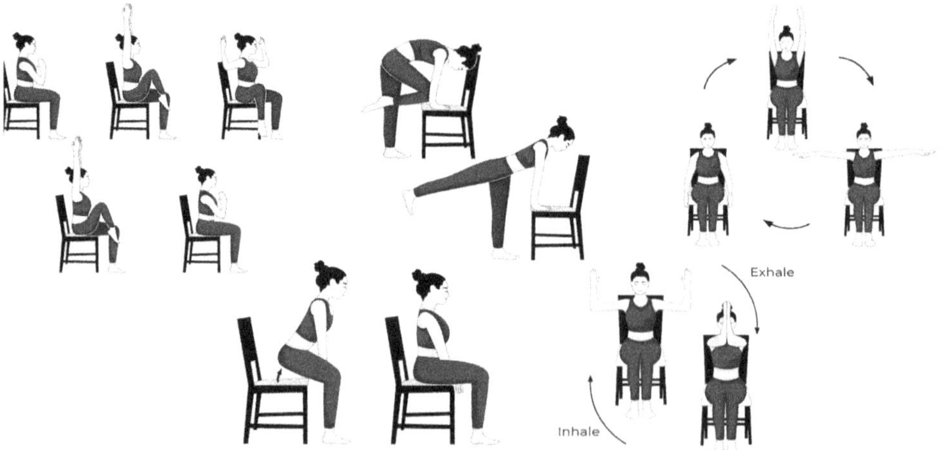

Exhale

Inhale

Third: Revitalizing Foundation – Feet and Ankles, Hip Openers

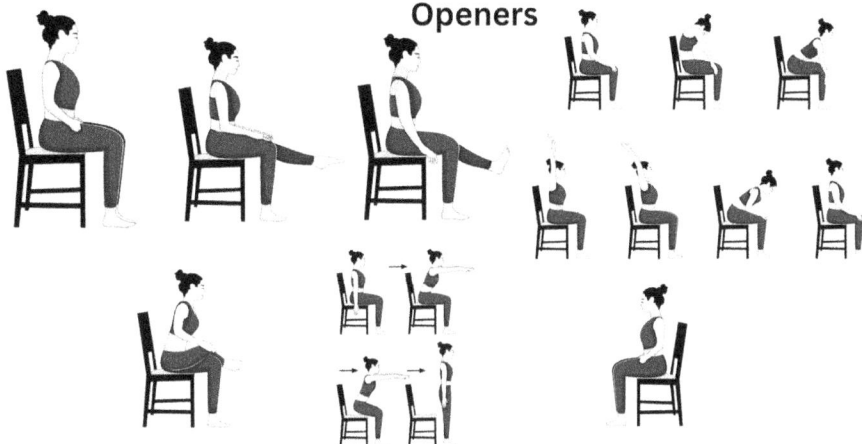

References

Anne, H. (2019, June 17). *7 reasons why warmup and proper breathing is important for yoga*. Simplejoy.co.uk. https://simplejoy.co.uk/2019/06/17/warmup-and-breathing-in-yoga/.

Better Health Channel. (2012). *Ageing — muscles bones and joints*. Vic.gov.au. https://www.bett erhealth.vic.gov.au/health/conditionsandtreatments/ageing-muscles-bones-and-joints.

Bisht, H. (2022, September 28). *Benefits of bhramari pranayama and how to do it*. PharmEasy Blog. https://pharmeasy.in/blog/health-fitness-benefits-of-bhramari-pranayama-and-how-to-do-it/.

Burgin, T. (2012, May 11). *Dirga pranayama*. Yoga Basics. https://www.yogabasics.com/practice/dirga-pranayama/.

Burgin, T. (2021, June 8). *Sama vritti pranayama (box breath or equal breathing)*. Yoga Basics. https://www.yogabasics.com/practice/sama-vritti-pranayama/

Chair yoga for seniors, beginner friendly | Living Maples. (2023, February 12). Living Maples. https://livingmaples.com/mag/chair-yoga-for-seniors/#:~:text=hatha%20yoga.

Cronkleton, E. (2018, August 15). *How to breathe and ways to breathe better*. Healthline. https://www.healthline.com/health/how-to-breathe#stronger-diaphragm.

Excellence in Fitness. (n.d.). *How long does it take for older adults to build muscle?* Excellence in Fitness. Retrieved February 10, 2023, from https://www.excellenceinfitness.com/blog/how-long-does-it-take-for-older-adults-to-build-muscle.

Guillemets, T. (2002). *Yoga quotes (hatha yoga, asanas, etc.).* Www. quotegarden.com. https://www.quotegarden.com/yoga.html.

Living Maples. (2022, July 2). *Chair yoga for seniors, beginner friendly.* Living Maples. https://livingmaples.com/mag/chair-yoga-for-seniors.

Manning, M. (2021). Exercise the Gentle Way with Chair Yoga for Seniors. *Sixty and Me.* https://sixtyandme.com/benefits-of-chair-yoga-for-seniors/#:~:text=wonderful%20health%20benefits.

MPH, C. A., MD, & MD, N. R. (2021, December 6). *Yoga for weight loss: Benefits beyond burning calories.* Harvard Health. https://www.health.harvard.edu/blog/yoga-for-weight-loss-benefits-beyond-burning-calories-202112062650.

Nunez, K. (2020, May 15). *Pranayama benefits for physical and emotional health.* Healthline. https://www.healthline.com/health/pranayama-benefits#less-stress.

Pal, G. K., Agarwal, A., Shamanna, K., Pal, P., & Nanda, N. (2014). Slow yogic breathing through right and left nostril influences sympathovagal balance, heart rate variability, and cardiovascular risks in young adults. *North American Journal of Medical Sciences*, 6(3), 145. https://www.ncbi.nlm.nih.gov/pmc/articles/PMC3978938/#:~:text=%5B16%2C17%2C18%5D,the%20representative%20of%20parasympathetic%20activation.

Pat's Chair Yoga. (n.d.). *FAQs.* Pat's Chair Yoga. Retrieved February 10, 2023, from https://patschairyoga.com/faqs/.

Pizer, A. (2020a, June 3). *Step by step instructions for dirga pranayama three-part breath.* Verywell Fit. https://www.verywellfit.com/three-part-breath-dirga-pranayama-3566762.

Pizer, A. (2020b, June 30). *Easily learn ujjayi breath to deepen your yoga practice*. Verywell Fit. https://www.verywellfit.com/ocean-breath-ujjayi-pranayama-3566763.

Ryt, A. P. (2022). 10 chair yoga poses you can do at home. *Verywell Fit*. https://www.verywellfit.com/chair-yoga-poses-3567189#:~:text=Better%20Posture

Senior Lifestyle. (2020, February 12). *Top 10 chair yoga positions for seniors [infographic]*. Senior Lifestyle. https://www.seniorlifestyle.com/resources/blog/infographic-top-10-chair-yoga-positions-for-seniors.

Stelter, G. (2020, May 29). *7 yoga poses you can do in a chair*. Healthline. https://www.healthline.com/health/fitness-exercise/chair-yoga-for-seniors#Seated-Forward-Bend-(Paschimottanasana).

Stump, M. (2017, June 16). *Yoga and its many benefits*. Lifespan. https://www.lifespan.org/lifespan-living/yoga-and-its-many-benefits.

University of Michigan Health. (n.d.). *Diaphragmatic breathing for GI patients*. Www.uofmhealth.org. https://www.uofmhealth.org/conditions-treatments/digestive-and-liver-health/diaphragmatic-breathing-gi-patients.

WebMD. (2021, October 25). *What to know about alternate-nostril breathing*. WebMD. https://www.webmd.com/balance/what-to-know-about-alternate-nostril-breathing.

Wu, Y., Johnson, B. T., Acabchuk, R. L., Chen, S., Lewis, H. K., Livingston, J., Park, C. L., & Pescatello, L. S. (2019). *Yoga as antihypertensive lifestyle therapy: A systematic review and meta-analysis. Mayo Clinic Proceedings*, *94*(3). https://doi.org/10.1016/j.mayocp.2018.09.023.

Yoga for Seniors: benefits, poses, chair yoga | Lifeline Canada. (2023, September 21). Lifeline. https://www.lifeline.ca/en/resources/yoga-for-seniors/#:~:text=back%20pain.

Zerbe, L. (2021, April 21). *Best Chair Yoga for Seniors: A 15 — Minute Routine to Reduce Pain & More* Dr. Axe. https://draxe.com/fitness/chair-yoga-for-seniors/.

Three Levels for Strength,
Posture, and Fitness
in Just 10 Minutes a Day

28 DAYS
OF
CHAIR EXERCISES
FOR WEIGHT LOSS

**99 ILLUSTRATED EXERCISES
ORGANIZED INTO 28 ROUTINES**

Ottie Oz

Discover our Exclusive Joint & Ankle Sequences!

Scan QR code

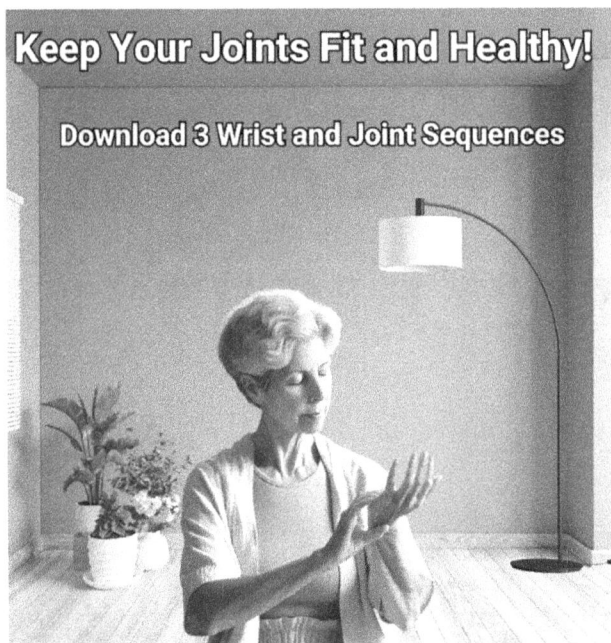

Keep Your Joints Fit and Healthy!

Download 3 Wrist and Joint Sequences

Elevate your mobility and ease discomfort with our expertly designed sequences. Perfect for enhancing flexibility, reducing pain, or adding mindfulness to your day, these sequences are the ultimate upgrade to your wellness routine. Start feeling the difference today!

Introduction

How old would you be if you didn't know how old you are?
— Reverend Clarence H. Wilson

We are living in an ever-changing world, and one positive change seen in recent times is the level of interest in longevity. There is also increasing interest in the mature population regarding leading a physically healthier life into the later years of life.

Recent population figures indicate that there are over 750 million people alive today over the age of 65 (United Nations, 2022) , more than at any other time in recorded history. To put this into context, this is nearly six times higher than in 1950. During this same period, the world's life expectancy has also risen sharply. In 1950, globally, the average person was expected to live 47 years. Today, this figure sits at 71 years (Dattani et al., 2023). Someone born 70 years ago will have been born shortly after the Second World War—before telephones and even televisions were in every home, before man walked on the moon, before computers and the internet became mainstream, and before mobile phones were even an idea. By the opposite measure, someone born today will almost certainly live to see the new century—2100.

The rise in life expectancy and the number of older adults still with us can be attributed to many reasons, one of which is how many more of us are leading relatively active lifestyles. For many seniors, living an active lifestyle is not necessarily something new. They, after all, grew up in a time when children would generally spend their free time playing outside rather than inside.If you are fortunate enough to have lived to a great age, what may have changed since these years is the ease with which you are able to execute these physical activities. For some, the struggles might be limited to specific body parts and activities. For others, it may even be more severe and interfere with everyday life, like getting out of bed or keeping balance while on their feet.

With advances in the understanding of the human body and ways in which we can treat aging muscles and body parts, the increasingly difficult future many older citizens face (especially with regard to the feeling of the body failing them) need not be your future. What if this future can be avoided by simply using an everyday item that is probably already in your possession and that you already use every day?

In this book, we will explore how the simple four-legged chair can be used to turn back your body's clock. Through targeted exercises, you will soon rebuild withering muscles, restore balance, and slowly but surely gain confidence, leading to an improved quality of life. We will also look into the benefits of remaining active as you age, provide a step-by-step guide as to how to execute chair exercises, assist you in building and maintaining your exercise plan and routine, address weight management, and ultimately leave you leading your best life possible.

Being Active and Embracing Fitness at Any Age

Those who think they have not time for bodily exercise will sooner or later have to find time for illness.

— Edward Stanley

As alluded to earlier, the portion of the population living into their 60s and beyond has never been greater. It is one thing to be alive at that age, and it is a completely different take if you are still able to live life during these years. For many, to continue living life and enjoying everything they hold dear, it is of great importance that people look after their physical well-being as their bodies morph.

Before we delve deeper into the topic, it's so good to see the significant impact of exercise on older individuals. It's not uncommon to see people in their 60s, 70s, and even 80s achieving incredible physical activity results. For instance, within the running clubs, numerous members actively participate in marathons and ultramarathons in their later years. Or they are playing tennis with friends. This challenges common perceptions, proving that an active lifestyle is more than just for the younger generation. It's very pleasing to see the older population being active—taking up sports they had never done before and excelling at them! These examples are powerful testaments to the possibilities that await when one embraces an active lifestyle, regardless of age. I'm sure you've heard that before that age; it's just a number, right? People have varying levels of mobility, but fortunately, you can easily modify exercises to suit individual needs. You can perform many of them while sitting and still reap the benefits.

While not every senior is destined to perform extreme feats at the age groups mentioned above, it is no longer uncommon to see them taking part in physical activities like surfing or squash weekly with people half their age or even newsworthy when folks in their 70s summit great mountain peaks. These active lifestyles continue to play a significant role in the changing face of mature people.

No longer is it considered the norm for seniors to spend the day alternating between the bed, the couch, and the seat on the porch, with their bodies slowly shriveling and muscles and tendons wasting away. Sure, not many are as spry as they once were, but no physical activity (or attempts at it) should be discounted. Not only that, but it is now commonplace to see an older person leading an independent lifestyle.

Being able to maintain these lifestyles is but one benefit of regular physical activity and exercise. Tying into the topic of longevity and more active lifestyles, research has also shown the medical benefits of regular physical activity. Studies have specifically focused on the role that active lifestyles play in lowering the chances of contracting heart diseases, diabetes, strokes, and many forms of cancer (World Health Organization, 2018). These diseases are also among the leading causes of death throughout the world, so one can see how increased levels of physical activity across the population have likely led to people living longer lives.

Over the years, a number of studies have also focused on the positive mental benefits of physical activity. One such recent study showed that the risk of depression among older adults, whether they had chronic pain or not, was lower when they performed moderate physical activity regularly (Laird et al., 2023). This specific study included those who already suffer from chronic pain in order to eliminate criticism of bias in previous studies (where healthier individuals made up the observed subjects).

It has furthermore been illustrated how physical activity in the elderly unlocks key benefits when it comes to movement and improved cognitive function (better command of one's own body, such as factors relating to strength and flexibility). The same study also saw improved concentration and more focused relaxation (Picorelli et al., 2014).

There are, of course, many rollover benefits as well, like social benefits. For example, a golfer who is able to remain active within his society will be able to maintain his long-standing friendships a lot better should he remain capable of meeting his golfing friends weekly for a round and enjoying a drink thereafter.

The U.S. Department of Health and Human Services (2018) lists many more benefits of regular physical activity: improved sleep, reduced levels of anxiety, and reduced blood pressure in the short term. In addition to the abovementioned benefits, in the long term, the following benefits are listed: balance and coordination (important for avoiding falls), improved bone health, and healthier weight management (which we will explore in depth in a later chapter).

Suppose you have time to go through the source material for many of the studies mentioned above. In that case, it will become clear that they do not necessarily always list what physical activity was done. You, as someone to whom chair exercises are clearly a topic of interest, may then be left wondering if any of the above applies to chair exercises. The good news is that they are.

Owing to their versatile nature, chair exercises indeed hold many benefits. Some of these include the following:

- **Convenience:** It can be done anywhere and at any time.
- **Inclusivity:** Anyone who is able to sit upright under their own power will be able to do chair exercises.

- **Muscle building:** This is not just limited to the arms but rather the entire body.

- **Cardio workouts are possible:** There are truly exercises that target a variety of facets of physical health.

- **Improved mobility:** Perhaps this is what many will be most familiar with (when picturing rehabilitation patients).

Now that we've looked through some of the benefits of physical activity and chair exercises specifically, it is also important that we examine some of the common misconceptions and false narratives surrounding the older population and exercise. The foremost of these is the most frequent excuse: "I am too old" (or a variation thereof). There are endless examples of amazing elderly folks doing amazing things. You only need to head over to the Guinness World Records website and type "oldest" in the search bar to find some of these (from the oldest active mechanic to the oldest person to perform a headstand).

Having previously been an easy escape route, the claims that all exercise worsens current physical ailments (such as arthritis) have been studied in depth and debunked through numerous undertakings. The Mayo Clinic (2023) even explicitly prescribes exercise as an essential tool in fighting arthritis, citing range of motion, strengthening, and aerobic exercises as key.

How often through our lives have we heard elder relatives or friends state that they are too limited in what they can do? From not being able to stand for extended periods to having limited mobility, these are not excuses that can be generally used for chair exercises. The exercises in this book are crafted to accommodate a wide range of situations. Bundled under this branch of excuses, many of us are of the belief that our risk of falling increases if we take part in physical activities. While this might hold some truth for activities that involve standing, chair exercises, for the most part, eliminate this aspect.

Lastly, there's the excuse that just about every person has used at least once in their life: "I don't have time." This is a simple case of finding your *why*, a topic to which we have dedicated an entire chapter in this book. Without your *why*, it is highly unlikely that your exercise program will be sustainable. This will, of course, vary from person to person, but the importance remains. "I don't have enough time" only applies if your grander goals are not a priority.

Now that we have had a look at some of the benefits and challenges that many face, we can dive into some other aspects. Exercise is a good launching pad, but to successfully achieve an improved quality of life, it needs to be coupled with a smarter diet and, better yet, weight management.

Managing Weight Loss with Exercises and Savvy Food Choices

Exercise is king. Nutrition is queen.
Put them together and you've got a kingdom.

— Jack Lalanne

"Lose 20 pounds in 3 weeks" is how a typical infomercial starts, making promise after promise on the benefits of their new "miracle" product, which will apparently leave you looking and feeling younger than ever before. Now and again, they will even feature a so-called expert or have a celebrity (or pseudo-celebrity) endorse the product. Have you ever wondered why these infomercials rarely, if ever, feature anyone with a Ph.D. or Dr. in their title? This is no coincidence, as a doctor is required to take a Hippocratic oath, and should they knowingly mete out bad advice or suggest treatments not based on and rooted in medical science, there is a good chance they'll never be able to practice again.

What happens to the aforementioned experts or celebrities if the product is found to not yield all the benefits promised? Nothing. What many of these miracle products fail to mention is that behind the scenes, all those who consumed the product were more than likely also put on an exercise program as well as an adjusted and controlled eating plan. Imagine the world we could be living in if regular exercise and healthier eating plans were pushed to the front and center of the public psyche.

This book follows the approach that calls for a combination of both exercises and a healthy diet to create what is called a calorie deficit for weight loss (or maintenance). The concept of calorie deficits is very simple: Is your body using everything you put into it? If you eat and drink more calories than you use throughout a given day, you'll have a calorie surplus. A sustained surplus will result in weight gain, while a sustained deficit over time will result in weight loss. On the whole, small differences should balance out in the long term.

It is also of utmost importance that we start by acknowledging that, in order to continue functioning optimally, the body does actually need calories. So it goes without saying that you should not deprive yourself of food or drink. We will just be seeking to eat and drink in a healthier manner and in the quantities we need. When you exercise more, you will require additional calories. The converse holds true when you move less.

These required quantities vary based on a broad number of factors. The best estimates have the average adult male requiring 2,500 kcal, while the average female requires 2,000 kcal daily (NHS, 2021). Some factors alluded to earlier that cause variations in requirements include age, weight, height, and how much exercise the individual does. For individuals 51 years of age and older, it is estimated that this figure could range between 2,000 and 2,800 kcal for males and between 1,600 and 2,200 kcal for females (Callahan et al., 2020). And yet again, I want to reiterate that it depends on the person and their circumstances.

There are two important factors I would like to point out before we continue. Firstly, as with most long-term and sustainable lifestyle changes, you will not be expected to go cold turkey and immediately and completely overhaul your diet. And secondly, while the subject of calorie reduction can sound overly scientific and complicated, it definitely need not be. Sure, there are definitely more precise ways of determining the number of calories you need. And yes, there are definitely more scientific ways to go about logging how many calories you consume daily. However, many find that lifestyle changes fail when the person feels like it becomes a chore to keep it going, which would be the case if it involves frequent and overcomplicated calculations.

We are therefore looking at easier and more practical ways in which we can avoid this. And, thankfully, there are means available. You could think of it in terms of an artistic interpretation of a tree by two artists. One artist might use a fine paintbrush and intricately and meticulously paint each branch and leaf of the tree. Another might use a broader brush and simply paint the brown base of the tree and a green circle on top. From a few feet away, most people will easily be able to identify the latter as a tree, despite the lack of care taken in producing the painting.

The same goes for how we will approach the concept of creating a calorie deficit. Let's not focus on day-to-day calorie counting but rather on creating the best possible overall picture with our available means. There are many natural and easy ways of reducing calories, and the simplest way of doing this is to create a healthier eating plan containing more whole foods.

What exactly are whole foods? While there are no strict accreditations or certificates that are issued identifying them, whole and unprocessed foods are foods that are sold as close as possible to their natural state. The next time you're at the grocery store, you should be easily able to identify them. They are commonly unpackaged (or minimally packaged) and free of additives. Unfortunately, there has been a great drive toward convenience over the past few decades, to the point where many associate whole foods with blandness. Again, this is certainly not the case, as spices and healthier condiments form part of cleaner diets.

So, what exactly does a healthy and balanced diet look like? In keeping with the latest scientific medical findings, the USDA (2020) recommends the following (with some examples listed):

- Consume more whole and unprocessed fruits and vegetables (rich in vitamins, fiber, antioxidants, potassium, manganese, iron, etc.):
  - apples
  - bananas
  - oranges
  - blueberries
  - strawberries
  - avocado
  - broccoli
  - carrots
  - kale
- Consume more whole grains (loaded with carbohydrates and fiber):
  - steel-cut oats
  - brown rice
  - quinoa
  - whole wheat pasta and wraps
  - certain breads (e.g., Ezekiel bread) in moderation
- Consume more lean meats and pulses (high in protein):
  - eggs
  - lean beef
  - chicken breasts
  - salmon

- ◆ tuna
- ◆ lentils
- ◆ chickpeas
- ◆ beans

- ✘ Include healthy oils (for healthy fats):
  - ◆ olive oil
  - ◆ canola oil

- ✘ Include dairy (the less processed, the better):
  - ◆ low-fat milk
  - ◆ cheese
  - ◆ yogurt

While not outwardly encouraged, the occasional consumption of processed foods and drinks does not necessarily cancel out all progress. Simply try as far as possible to hop back onto the wagon as soon as possible. It should also be noted that there are varying degrees of food processing. It is advisable to avoid the most processed products (referred to as ultra-processed). Some common examples of ultra-processed foods include mass-produced bread, most mass-produced cereals, chips, most carbonated drinks, yogurts with fruit flavoring, and mass-produced meats.

So, what are some of the changes we can look to implement? Firstly, perhaps rethink the manner in which you consume food. Combining foods into a solitary dish is nothing new. Dishes like curries and stews have been around for millennia and can pretty much be found across every continent and in every culture. For the purpose of adding fruits and vegetables to your diet, why not consider having more homemade smoothies in summer and soups in winter? Consider using wraps instead of bread, honey instead of sugar, iced tea instead of carbonated drinks, oats instead of cornflakes, and chicken breasts and lean beef or pork steak cuts instead of chicken and beef burgers, sausages, and ham. While it might seem difficult to navigate at first, you'll soon pick it up.

By now, many of you will already be wondering, *How do I know how big a portion is?* While these are obviously not scientifically accurate to a tee, there are a few simple unofficial rules of thumb you can use as a cheat sheet to get an idea of portion sizes:

- **Open palm:** One portion of meats and other proteins
- **Closed fist:** One portion of fruits and vegetables
- **Cupped palm:** One portion of grains (and other carbohydrates)
- **Thumb:** One portion of oils (and other fats)

By replacing the heavily processed foods you may currently be consuming with more of the above, you are already creating a calorie deficit relative to your current status quo. By adding regular exercise to the equation, the benefits multiply. To further illustrate the effect of exercise on the body's use of calories, consider roughly how much you need to exercise to "cancel out" the following commonly consumed goods:

- 1 can of soda equals 26 minutes of walking or 13 minutes of running.
- 1 standard chocolate bar equals 42 minutes of walking or 22 minutes of running.
- 1 standard bag of chips equals 31 minutes of walking or 16 minutes of running.
- 1 iced cinnamon bun equals 1 hour and 17 minutes of walking or 40 minutes of running.

It's not advisable to adopt an attitude where you bargain with yourself—like drinking a can of soda with the justification of walking the dog later. This approach rarely works. I echo Dr. Yoni Freedhoff's sentiment that you can't outrun your fork. I've tried it myself and failed a few times. A balanced approach is key: both exercise and a healthy diet need to become integral parts of your life.

The final point of discussion in this chapter pertains to whether or not chair exercises can effectively be used for weight loss. The simple answer is yes. As long as you are using up energy and burning more calories (which you do even by simply moving or even more so when exercising at a high intensity) than what you have consumed, you will be able to lose weight. This obviously differs from person to person, but in any event, you are definitely better off doing some exercises than none at all.

Hopefully, you have a better understanding by now of the principles of weight loss and management. In the end, it is as simple as asking yourself, "Am I using more calories than I'm putting into my body?" If yes, you will create a calorie deficit. Sustain this over a period of time, and you should notice weight loss.

Finding Your Why, Committing to New Routines, And Achieving Your Fitness Goals

He who has a why to live can bear almost any how.
— Friedrich Nietzsche

Many diets fail. Understanding why they do can be a key in our journey toward a healthier lifestyle. The reasons for these failures often come down to a few missteps. One major pitfall is setting unrealistic goals or not setting them at all. Getting caught up in ambitious targets that are not feasible in the short term is easy. Another common issue is focusing excessively on calorie counting. This can lead to an unhealthy obsession rather than a balanced approach to eating.

However, the most significant oversight is failing to recognize that adopting a healthier lifestyle is a long-term commitment. It involves gradually and consistently replacing unhealthy habits with healthier ones—creating new routines. This isn't just about a temporary change in diet; it's about embarking on a journey to discover what works best for you personally, understanding that this process takes time and patience.

Finding your "why" is a crucial part of this journey. I learned it the hard way. Like many, I couldn't wrap my head around a healthy lifestyle for quite a long time. I found myself trying different diets; some of them were strict ones. I was "on a diet" very often. It was almost "my thing." Admittedly, they have offered short-term solutions but never lasted long enough if I managed to get through them. You might assume that after more than several failed attempts, I would realize something is wrong and that these diets don't' really work. Yet, it took me long and painful years to realize this approach wasn't practical or effective.

My good friend's journey to a healthier lifestyle was inspiring and surprising. We used to be very active kids—constantly on the move. The afternoons were spent playing volleyball with classmates and neighborhood kids. Summer holidays were filled with endless bike rides and swims in the lake. As time went on, our paths crossed less and less.

While I was increasingly engrossed in music school and spent most of my time in classes and doing homework, she explored different passions. She had a knack for languages. She spent most of her time buried in books and taking part in language clubs. This intellectual pursuit, though enriching, meant less time for physical activities for both of us. The active lifestyle of our childhood slowly faded into the background. Our diet, increasingly distant from any notion of healthiness, followed suit.

As time passed, we transformed from wide-eyed kids into all-knowing teenagers—in our minds, the masters of the universe. And then it arrived—exams, school graduation, university applications.

We've been accepted at different universities in separate towns, yet we stayed connected. Despite our busy academic lives, we met roughly every six months. The first time I saw her after we parted ways, I was taken aback. She lost a significant amount of weight. She said that she had joined a weight loss club and followed a strict diet for six weeks. However, during our day together, I couldn't help but notice her indulgence in sugary treats—a diet I couldn't help thinking, with a touch of irony, that I could get on board with.

The next time we met, she appeared different from just half a year before. She was devastated that she had regained the weight she lost and added more. This cycle continued for a few years. Our meetings became less frequent, but she dropped a bombshell during one of our phone conversations—she was training for a half-marathon. The news was more than surprising; it was astounding.

I attended her first event, as I wanted to be there for her.

I couldn't wait to hear what had happened. A half-marathon?! She shared her turning point with me when we sat down to catch up. After one particularly disheartening episode with junk food, she felt a physical and emotional low. She hit the bottom with her dieting. She realized that she wanted a change—a lasting change.

She started with simple walks. They challenged her more than expected. But instead of discouraging her, these difficulties fueled her determination.

Slowly, her short walks turned into longer ones, taking shapes as short runs and, eventually, long-distance running. She confided that her mindset had shifted: it was no longer about restricting herself but about nourishing her body and mind with healthy food to support her new passion. She had accidentally stumbled upon her "why," and it was running. To be able to train and take part in all sorts of running competitions, she had to take care of her body.

As I listened to her story, I felt a surge of happiness for her. I did. She had found her purpose, her motivation—her "why." And as for me, I realized I was still on my journey, searching for my own.

That first half-marathon was a milestone. She may not have set a record, but her personal accomplishment was immense. She had found her "why."

I am well aware that this is an example of extreme proportions, but it can be applied to any situation and any *why*. There are limitless examples, and they will almost certainly differ from person to person. For many, the reasoning for wanting to stay healthy might be as simple as living to see and play with their grandchildren. It may be to remain fit enough to continue playing a sport they enjoy participating in. It may be for more personal reasons, like remaining confident in their movements or even remaining confident in their appearance.

As much as there is no one-size-fits-all for finding your *why*, there is also no single approach that will guarantee your successful journey to a healthier you. For each person, this journey will look different— different in terms of weight goals, in terms of time taken, and in how they go about reaching them. That being said, there are some general guidelines given by the CDC (2022) as to how to go about achieving sustainable weight loss:

- **Make a commitment:** Write down these goals, and make sure they are visible daily.

- **Take stock of where you are:** Write down your current diet and when and why you waver from healthy eating (e.g., when moody, pressed for time, or around certain people).

- **Set realistic goals:** You might find it better to have both short-term goals (exercise for 100 minutes a week, replace soda with sugar-free iced tea, or cut down your portions of bread) and long-term goals (continue playing golf, continue to be able to go shopping by yourself, or even get fit enough to summit a specific mountain). Also, be realistic, specific (not just "lose weight" but rather "lose 10 lbs in one month"), and flexible (forgiving) in your goal settings.

- **Identify supporters:** Find like-minded people (e.g., family, friends, or groups) and resources (e.g., social media pages with encouraging messages, healthy recipes, or newsletters notifying you of nearby events you might enjoy) that will aid your journey to wellness.

- **Monitor progress:** Remember to take stock regularly. One day or a few days of failure doesn't spell defeat. Don't neglect to celebrate your successes and readjust goals as needed (e.g., increase your exercise minutes or cut down further on sugar if you started off only cutting down slightly).

Tend to focus on your long-term goals of eating healthy and exercising enough to continue doing what you enjoy, and weight management is kind of just a by-product of that lifestyle. I have found a simple analogy for this in the form of stock analysis.

Let's say you own a company. If you were to follow the movement of your company's stock price over five years, you may have observed its upward trend from $5 per share to $20 on a graphic representation for the five-year period. Most would consider this a success in the long term, right? Now consider if you were to zoom in on just the first year of activity. You may have seen fluctuations where the first six months may have read $5, $6, $7, $5, $6, and $6 despite you continuing to put resources into the company. Many people might stop here and consider the investment a failure, as the stock price only grew by $1. Over the next six months, the price might change again: $7, $9, $8, $11, $12, and closing on $12 for year one. By now, most would consider this a success as the investment more than doubled, correct?

If you zoom in deep enough, you'll find a two-week period where you gained 5 lbs. Yet, if you zoom out for that month, you remain constant. Always remember the bigger picture, and always keep your focus on the long-term goal. Continue to "put in the resources" (i.e., exercises and healthy eating), and in the bigger picture, probably without even realizing it, the weight will manage itself.

Now that you're aware of the *why* and the long-term outlook, I bet you're itching to know how you go about practically implementing chair exercises into your routine. Here are some tips that I myself and others have found helpful in starting new exercise routines:

- **Experiment:** Try out different exercise routines at different times of the day (morning vs. evening) for short periods of time (like one week) to see which works best.

- **Consistency**: If you're looking to have your healthy eating and exercise become a habit (without giving it much thought), you'll need to start by having it as a routine (scheduled frequently, intentionally, and repeatedly). The best way is to practice these things daily.

- **Start as simple as possible**: Every single person who has ever accomplished what you consider to be incredible had to start somewhere. The hardest part will be to show up on that chair—the rest will be history.

- **Get a workout buddy or group:** It is always a lot harder to cancel if you know your no-show is going to disappoint others.

- **Prepare:** Make things as easy as possible for yourself. Set out your workout clothing the night before, and set your chair in plain view so that there's no avoiding it. I, for example, often roll out my yoga mat next to my bed before I retire to bed. This way, there is no avoiding it the next morning.

- **Allow yourself flexibility:** No one is perfect. Simply do the best you can, and when you slip, get back into your routine as soon as possible. On days that you are struggling, try five minutes. Anything trumps nothing 100% of the time.

In closing, embarking on anything new in life is never easy. Additionally, the older you are, the harder this may be. But it is not impossible. The above will hopefully have provided you with enough tools to at least plan and start your journey. Knowing what has and has not worked for others is already as good a starting point as any. Throw in the fact that you should be able to tailor your goals as you need them, and you're all set to go.

Understanding Chair Exercises and the Benefits Of Them

The greatest miracle on earth is the human body.
It is stronger and wiser than you may realize,
and improving its ability to self-heal is within your control.

— Dr. Fabrizio Mancini

In this chapter, we will explore the benefits of chair exercises, as well as their impact on your body and why it's beneficial to practice them. By using these exercises regularly and sticking to a healthy eating plan, you will, without a doubt, soon start to see positive changes.

Neck rotation, extensions, and stretches help you improve posture, which worsens over the years, increase blood flow to the spinal cord, and relieve tension. Also, it boosts the strength of your neck. If you have a limited range of motion, it's important to remember not to force it. It's better to take it slowly and do it daily rather than once a week for an hour.

BENEFITS OF FRONT RAISES

Shoulder and chest muscles are strengthened through this isolation exercise, and definition on both the front and side of the shoulders will improve. This is vital for everyday life, as you use your shoulders to lift daily (e.g., lifting yourself out of a chair), and it has even been shown to reduce neck pain (Louw et al., 2017).

BENEFITS OF LATERAL RAISES

This specifically targets the deltoid's lateral and anterior heads. As with front raises, expect your shoulders to be strengthened and more flexible after doing these exercises regularly. With these raises, however, the left and right sides are worked independently, so discrepancies (between arms) can be corrected (Coratella et al., 2020). Doing these exercises regularly should also see your overall posture improve.

BENEFITS OF OVERHEAD PRESSES, BACK PRESSES, AND FRONT PRESSES

Overhead, back, and front presses are a great workout for your anterior deltoids, which are used whenever you perform an action that requires you to pull your shoulders back. An example would be when you need to reach for anything on a high shelf. Overhead presses are also probably one of the best exercises for improving your body's posture, even more so than lateral raises.

BENEFITS OF CORE STRENGTHENING EXERCISES

As explained earlier, the core muscles are made up of a group of muscles encompassing the entire torso. It consists of the abdomen muscles (front stomach), the obliques (internal and external side muscles), the transversus abdominis (the muscles surrounding the spine), the hips, and the lower back muscles. Some of the exercises that target the core include knee to elbow, extended leg raises, bicep curls, crossed arm crunches, and flutter kicks.

These exercises will play a pivotal role in improving the strength of your entire body; improving your balance, stability, and posture; assisting in making daily tasks like walking, getting out of bed, or standing up from a chair much easier; and assisting in reducing back and hip pain that plagues so many older adults.

BENEFITS OF SEATED CARDIO EXERCISES

Cardio exercises are an important part of any exercise routine as they get the heart pumping. By persistently doing these exercises, you will naturally decrease your resting heart rate and improve your heart muscles' ability to pump blood. In time, this will allow you to improve your exercise endurance. There are a host of other benefits for the body with all cardio exercises, which include lowering blood sugar, improving cholesterol, alleviating arthritic pains, and improving sleep and concentration.

Some examples of these exercises include seated jacks, lifts, leg lifts and twists, and chair running.

BENEFITS OF QUADRICEPS MUSCLE EXERCISES

Quadriceps refer to a group of four muscles (rectus femoris, vastus lateralis, vastus medialis, and vastus intermedius) running from the hips down to the front of the knee. The quadriceps are used in many of the daily activities we may take for granted. These include not only walking but also every time we either lower ourselves to sit or raise ourselves to stand up (e.g., using the bathroom). There are also benefits for the knees and hips, aiding posture, stability, and balance, as well as playing a role in decreasing the risk of osteoarthritis.

Some examples of these exercises include knee extensions, leg lifts, and sit-to-stand flow.

BENEFITS OF MODIFIED SUMO CHAIR
AND CHAIR SQUATS

The sumo chair and chair squat modifications are, without a doubt, one of the best exercises for your leg muscles. They target muscles ranging from the lower back and gluteal muscles through the hamstrings and quadriceps. As mentioned above, these muscles are used for a variety of day-to-day activities, so it would be in your best interest not to neglect strengthening them.

How to Use This Book and Frequently Asked Questions

Take the first step in faith.
You don't have to see the whole staircase,
just take the first step.

— Martin Luther King, Jr.

In this book, you will find three different warm-up routines. To avoid routine fatigue, you can keep rotating them before you embark on the day's exercises. There are 28 different chair exercise routines and a cooldown stretch routine to complete after each session. As a bonus, if you scan the QR code at the start of the book, you will be able to access additional sequences for your wrists and ankles.

HOW TO USE THIS BOOK

1. Select one of the three warm-up options.
2. Select one of the 28 exercise sequences.
3. Do the cooldown stretches routine.

It's as simple as one, two, three. While not absolutely necessary, it is suggested you try all the different warm-ups on consecutive days (e.g., on day one, do warm-up one; on day two, do warm-up two; on day three, do warm-up three), and do the same with the workouts. Doing this will help you figure out not only which warm-ups and workouts

How to Use This Book and Frequently Asked Questions

are agreeable to your body but also which ones you enjoy more. You may, for example, find a certain sequence to be of great benefit to your lower back, so you might want to do that sequence at least twice a week.

The exercises do not require you to have any other equipment except for a chair. For a start, you will only be using your own body weight. For more advanced fitness levels, you can use weights for exercises that require them. Even this, though, does not require you to go out and buy dumbbells, as you can simply use filled water bottles or even soup cans.

For beginners, it is also essential that you listen to your body, not only while doing the exercises but also before and after. Observe the effects certain sequences have on your body, and if you start to find the exercises are becoming too easy, you can add weights to them (and don't hesitate to drop them when the exercises become too tough midway through either).

FREQUENTLY ASKED QUESTIONS

If I have health issues, can I still practice?

If you have any health concerns, it might be best to consult your doctor or a physician before you start. While most older adults should be able to complete these exercises without problems, there are certain situations where certain individuals might not be able to do them.

What kind of chair do I need?

You need a sturdy chair with no arms. The absence of arms allows for greater flexibility in movement, and the key is to select a chair that remains steadfast throughout your exercise routine, providing stability without shifting or moving. Choose any regular, sturdy chair for exercises; steer clear of folding chairs or those with wheels.

Do I need any other special gear or equipment?

You also don't need any special clothing or gear. Any clothing that allows you freedom of movement to complete the exercises should be fine. For more advanced exercises, you can consider using dumbbells, water bottles, or soup cans.

How often should I do the chair exercises?

Most adults should aim for at least 150 minutes of moderately intense exercise per week (CDC, 2019). This can be split up into two or three sessions per week or even daily. The guideline of 150 minutes can be increased slowly and safely, should your fitness levels allow.

How do I know if chair exercises are right for me?

Seated workouts are especially useful for the elderly, those who have trouble standing for longer periods of time and moving around, and, generally, those who suffer from balance issues. They can also be used as part of a complementary existing routine (e.g. if you're an active tennis player, golfer, or hiker). Still, the best way to know if something is right for you is to try it out!

Warm-ups and cooldowns

It is highly advisable to do both if you're to ensure injury is avoided. Warm-ups assist in warming your body temperature and muscles up slowly and safely. It is also considered a good way of signaling to your brain that the body is about to embark on physical activity—a sort of mental heads-up. Cooldown stretches also play a role in absorbing the benefits of the exercise you've done. It also helps in bringing your heart rate back down to its pre-workout state.

What is the core, and how do I engage it?

The core refers to a group of muscles centered around the abdomen, pelvis, spine, and diaphragm. It plays a pivotal role in just about every exercise you do. Without being physically present and showing you, it can be a bit tricky to explain. I've found the easiest way is the same way I was taught: While lying on your back on a flat surface (like the floor or bed), place your thumbs slightly below either side of your belly. Now, give a light cough. The area that experienced rapid expansion and contraction is where you want to focus on *engaging*. Keep your thumbs in place, and imagine a small ball is being placed in between your thumbs. To engage your core, the aim would be to move this imaginary ball from between your thumbs toward your chest without moving the rest of your body. Tilt only the belly area in the direction of your chest, and you should feel those muscles *engaged*.

ROOM

So now you are all set to start with the exercises. You'll want to ensure your workout area is clear of any sharp objects and other matter that could get in the way and interfere with your routine or even injure you. Lastly, make sure the exercise space is as tidy and calming as possible to avoid distractions. And with that, you can start planning for your first chair exercise session.

Initiating Your Chair Exercise Journey: Correct Posture

As you embark upon chair exercises for weight loss journey, it is important to observe your posture. Your body's positioning and alignment play an important role in the effectiveness of each exercise. At the same time, it ensures your comfort and safety throughout the process.

Sit comfortably with your spine straight. Visualize an imaginary line gently pulling you upwards from the top of your head, facilitating spinal elongation.

Elevate your head, ensuring your gaze is directed straight ahead. This helps maintain a healthy neck posture while simultaneously allowing chest expansion, crucial for improved respiration.

Always slightly tuck your chink in. When we age, we tend to stick our neck out.

Gently roll your shoulders back and allow them to relax. Activate your core muscles by drawing your belly button towards your spine. This will assist as a stabilizing center for all movements.

Bend your knees at a comfortable 90-degree angle with your feet flat on the floor. Allow your arms to rest gently on your lap.

Do this posture check before each session, starting with your warm-up routines.

Progressing Through Your Chair Exercise Journey

Now that you've mastered the art of perfect posture, you're all set to embark on the chair exercise routines designed for each day. It's essential to understand that these exercises are structured to cater to everyone, starting from a basic level. Whether you're a beginner or looking to challenge yourself further, there's a clear path for progression.

Starting With the Basics

You will find a different set of exercises for each day. These sets are basic to ensure you can perform them safely and effectively, focusing on technique and alignment.

How to Increase Difficulty

As you grow more comfortable and seek to intensify your workouts, here's how to progress:

Level One: This is your starting point. Simply follow the exercises as outlined for each day. Repeat them three times, allowing two minutes to rest between each set.

Level One Variation: To add a bit of a challenge, repeat each exercise for 30 seconds. You can either use your body weight or introduce weights into the routine. Suitable options include light dumbbells, soup cans, or water bottles, depending on your comfort and capability. Repeat them three times, allowing two minutes to rest between the exercise sets.

Level Two: Repeat the sequence five times for an increased challenge, allowing yourself two minutes of rest between exercise sets. It will boost the intensity and help to build endurance.

Level Three: To push your limits further, complete the sequence seven times with two minutes of rest between the sets. This level is designed to maximize your strength and endurance gains.

You can experiment by reducing rest time between sets, increasing exercise intensity, adding weights to the exercises, increasing the repetition of the exercises, or maybe you prefer to set the timer and repeat each exercise for 20 seconds, later rising to 30 seconds, and to 45 seconds or a minute! This is your oyster. Observe how you feel, familiarize yourself with the exercises, and create your routines. My created routines are a starting point for you.

Remember, the key to a successful fitness journey is progressing at a pace that feels right for you. Each level is designed to build upon the last, gradually increasing in intensity to foster improvement without risking injury. Listen to your body, and don't rush the process. Consistency and patience are your best allies as you advance through the levels.

By incorporating weights or increasing the duration and repetition of the exercises, you'll enhance the challenge and keep your workouts exciting and varied. Keep pushing your boundaries, and celebrate every step forward in this journey toward health and vitality.

THREE WARM-UP AND COOLDOWN ROUTINES

Warm-ups are an important part of the workout. It prepares the body to exercise. It increases blood flow, warms the muscles, and makes them more flexible. This is to reduce the risk of injuries. Warm-ups also gradually raise the heart rate, which helps with muscle efficiency and improves overall performance. They also help with mental reparation. Your brain and body know what is coming next. Warming up your body is essential to any exercise routine, contributing to safety and effectiveness.

Please type into your browser
https://www.youtube.com/@ZenflowHub

Then, select 'Playlists,' where you will see several playlists available. Choose the one relevant to your book title, such as *28 Days of Chair Yoga for Seniors for Weight Loss.*

Or scan QR Code which will take you directly to the playlist

These videos are designed to assist you in performing the exercises detailed in this book. They serve as a valuable resource for checking your form or for additional clarification on the exercise techniques. The demonstrations include all exercises covered in the book, from warm-ups to main workout routines.

WARM-UP ONE

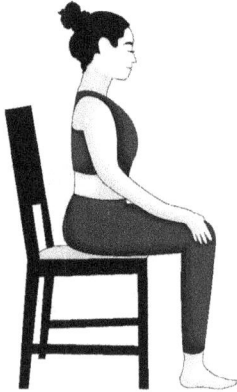

Before starting your warm-up routine, check your body's alignment first.

Sit and look up straight. Keep your chin ever so slightly tucked in.

Roll your shoulders back. Keep them relaxed. Lengthen your neck. Engage your core's stability. This is important for the exercise routines. Knees are bent at 90 degrees, and arms rest on your laps.

Neck Stretch

Keep your chin slightly tucked in. Turn your head gently to the right and then gently to the left. Hold the stretch for two to three seconds before moving your head to the opposite side. Repeat the same, moving your head up and down. Repeat three times in each direction—left, right, up, and down.

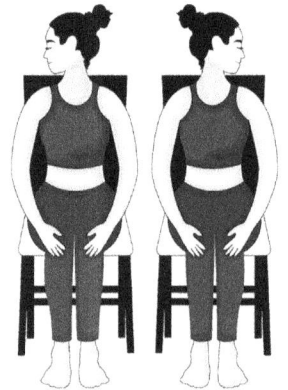

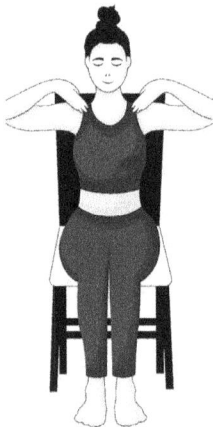

Shoulder Circles

Bring fingertips to shoulders—circle six to eight times in each direction. If you have limited mobility in your shoulders, then do only half of the circle.

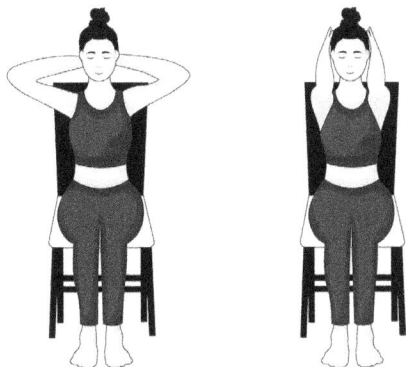

Shoulder Stretch

Bring your hands behind the head. Pull your elbows back as much as possible; imagine your shoulder blades having to keep a pencil between them. And then slowly move your elbows forward, trying to touch each other. Repeat the movement three to five times.

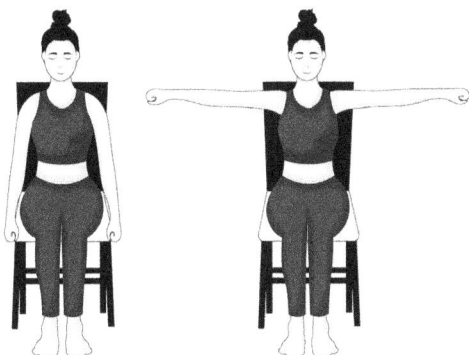

Lateral Arm Raises

Raise your arms parallel to the ground and at shoulder height, and lower them back to your sides. Feel your abdominal wall engaged, and don't hinge in the shoulders. Repeat the movement eight to ten times.

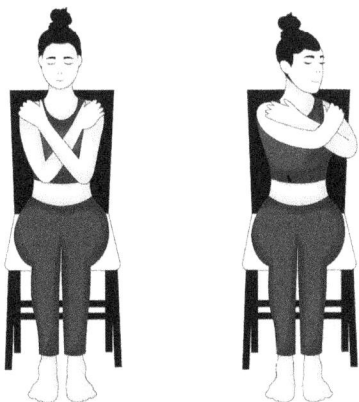

Upper Body Twist

Engage your core. Keep the chin slightly tucked in. Cross your arms on your chest and twist to the right. Return to the center, and then twist to the left. Alternate and repeat five to eight times.

Knee Extension

Extend your leg parallel to the floor or at the height that is comfortable for you. Feel your quadriceps muscles working on the front of the thigh. Repeat five to eight times, and then switch sides.

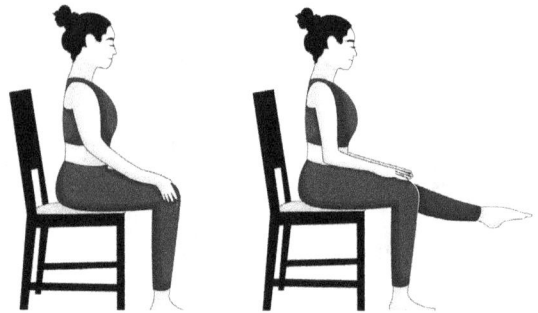

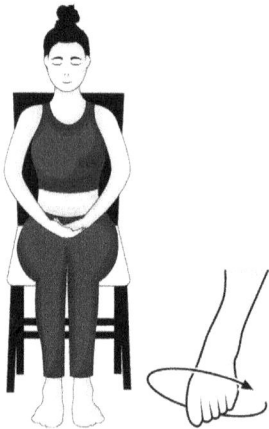

Ankle Circles

Lift your foot up a few inches from the floor, keeping your knee straight. Rotate the ankle one side three to five times, then in the opposite direction. Repeat the exercise with another leg.

Marching on the Spot

March on the spot, counting a total of 30 steps.

Now, you should be all warmed up and can continue your daily exercise routine. (Day 1, Day 2, etc.)

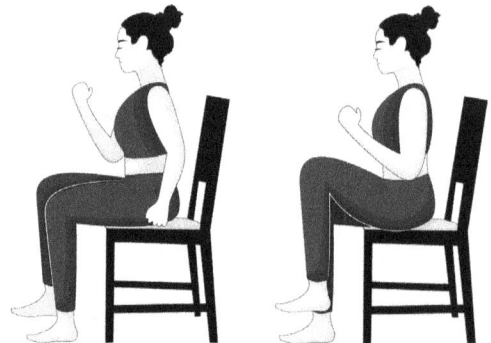

WARM-UP TWO

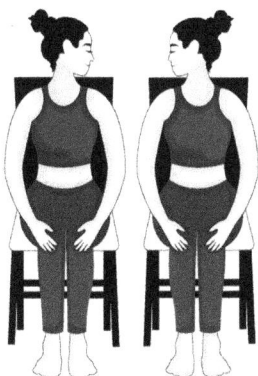

Neck Stretch

Keep your chin slightly tucked in. Turn your head gently to the right and then gently to the left. Hold the stretch for two to three seconds before moving your head to the opposite side. Repeat the same, moving your head up and down. Repeat three times in each direction—left, right, up, and down.

Shoulder Rolls

Keep the arms on your lap or next to you. Lift your shoulders and roll them back three times, then move them in the opposite direction.

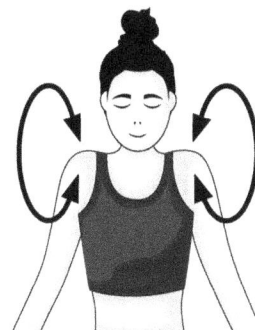

Chest Stretch

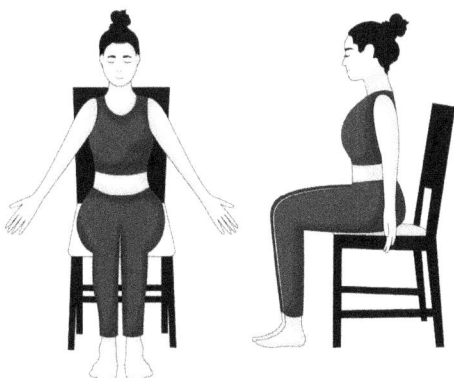

Begin by sitting tall, away from the back of the chair. Roll your shoulders back and down. Extend your arms to the sides, then gently press your chest forward and upward, savoring the stretch across your chest. Hold this position for five to eight seconds, and repeat it three to five times.

Upper Body Twist

Engage your core. Keep the chin slightly tucked in. Cross your arms on your chest and twist to the right. Return to the center, and then twist to the left. Alternate and repeat six to eight times.

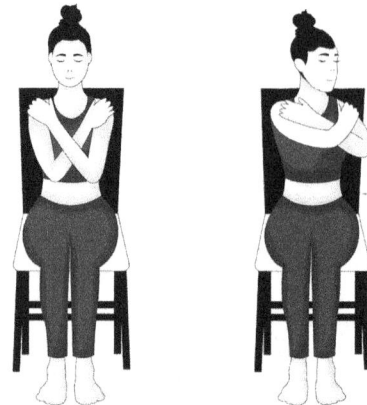

Flexing Foot

Lift your leg. Point the toes away from you. Pull the toes toward your chest and press the heel away. Repeat five to eight times before switching to the other leg.

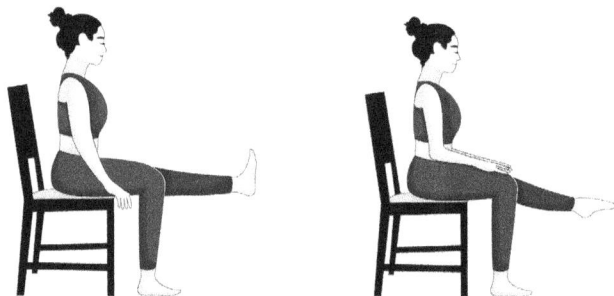

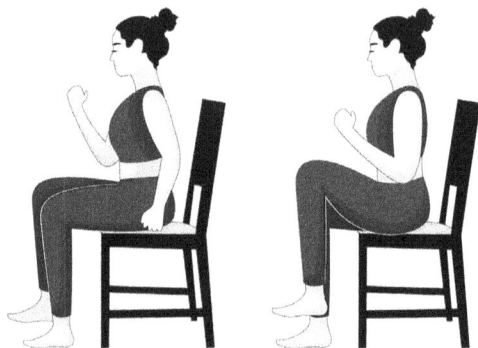

Marching on the Spot

March on the spot, counting a total of 30 steps.

WARM-UP THREE

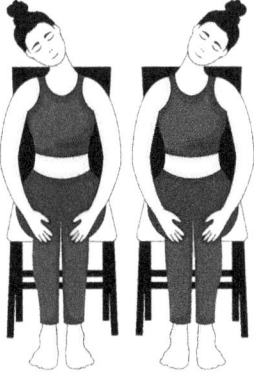

Neck Rolls

Start with small circles and roll your neck to the right side, slowly increasing the circle. The reverse—start with a big circle and get down to a small one, where you started. Repeat it once or twice.

Shoulder Shrugs

Inhale and raise your shoulders toward your earlobes. Keep your hands perpendicular to the floor throughout the exercise. Repeat six to eight times.

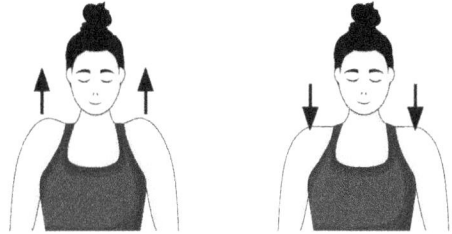

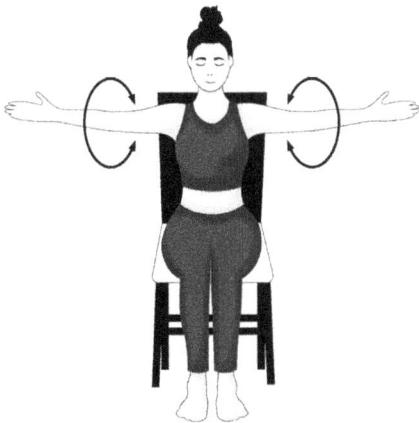

Arm Circles

Extend your arms to your sides. Keep them parallel to the floor at shoulder height. Slowly start to make small circles and keep increasing them. Complete five to eight moves in one direction and, when reversed, start with big circles and reduce them back to small circles.

Heel Raises

With your feet flat on the ground, lift your heels as high as you can off of the ground. You can do both legs or alternate. Repeat ten to fifteen times for each leg.

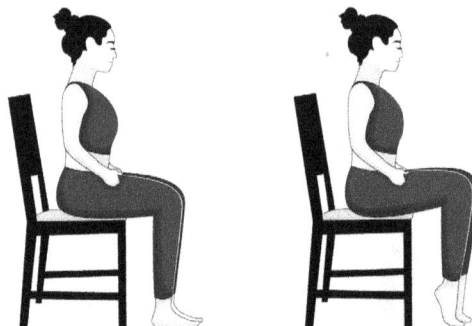

Front Punches

Keep your abdominals engaged. Bend your arms up so your wrists are by your shoulders. With control, slowly punch in front of, up, and across your body with one arm while slightly rotating your torso in the same direction. Return to the start position, then switch to the other arm. Alternate and repeat twenty times.

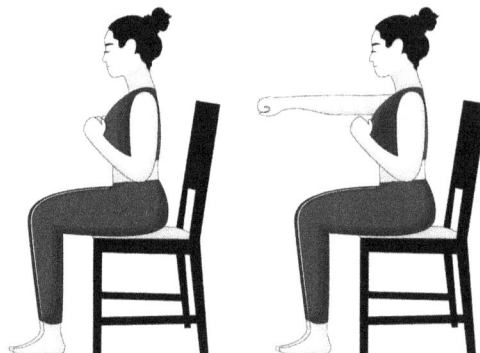

Overhead Punches

Bend your arms, and with control, slowly punch above your head with one arm. Fully straighten it, or as much as you can, and bring it down. Switch to the other arm. Alternate and repeat twenty times.

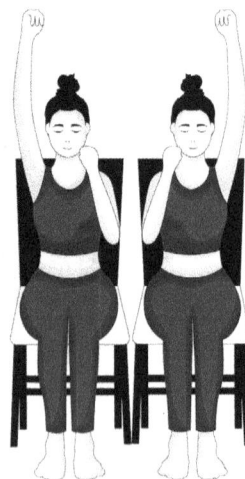

Run on the Spot

Instead of marching, run as fast as you can on the spot for 30 seconds.

Now, you should be all warmed up and can continue your daily exercise routine. (Day 1, Day 2, etc.)

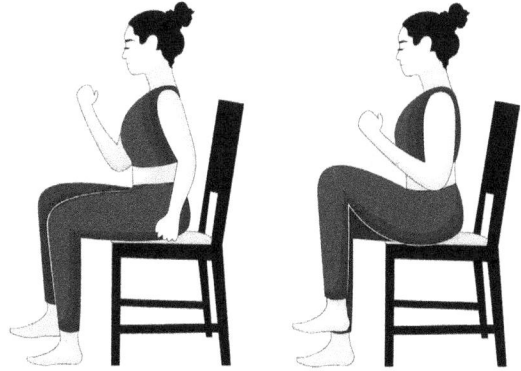

COOLDOWN ROUTINE

Cooldowns are a no less important part of the workout routine than warm-ups. Adding the cooldown routine to your workout helps your body slowly return to normal. Slowing down the heart rate and breathing reduces the risk of dizziness or fainting after intense exercise. Cooldowns are essential for easing muscle stiffness and soreness by helping to eliminate lactic acid buildup. They allow for muscle stretching, which enhances flexibility and prevents injuries. Cooldowns also give a moment for mental relaxation, signaling to your brain and body that the workout is complete.

Cross Body Shoulder Stretch

Take one arm and place it across your chest. Using your other hand, take the outer forearm of the arm that's across your body. Push that arm into your body to feel more of a stretch. Remain in the position for thirty seconds. Repeat with the other arm.

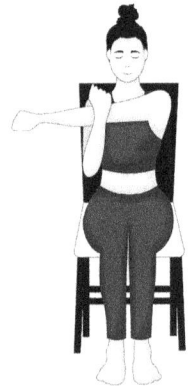

Triceps Stretch

When sitting down or standing up, roll your shoulders back.

Reach your right arm upward, then flex at the elbow to guide the right palm toward the middle of your back, placing your middle finger along your spine. Let your left hand guide your elbow toward the center and downward. Stay in this stretch for thirty seconds.Repeat it four times on each side.

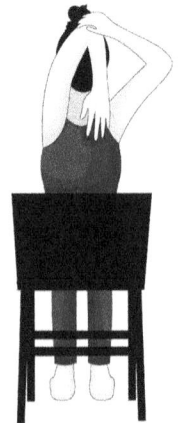

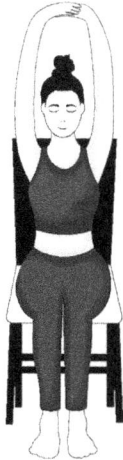

Upward Hand Stretch

Bring your arms in front and lengthen. Interlock your fingers with palms facing outside and raise your arms above your head. Keep fingers softly locked. Remain in the stretch for about three to four breaths. Repeat twice.

Forward Fold

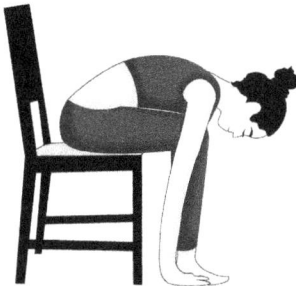

On the inhale, raise your arms up and gently stretch. On the exhale, take the arms toward your feet, with the torso resting on the thighs and chin close to the knees. Feel a stretch across your shoulders and back. To release, inhale, look up first, then raise your arms before returning to sit. Remain in the pose for two breaths or till you feel comfortable.

Note: If you have high blood pressure or difficulty breathing, you should not do this pose.

Hamstring Stretch

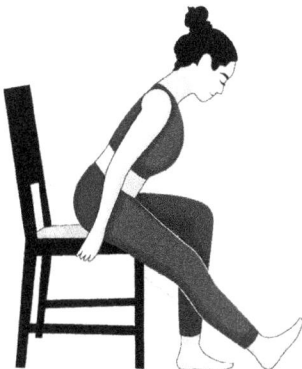

Sit closer to the front of the chair. Extend one leg in front of you, pulling the toes toward you. Lean as far as you can. Feel the hamstring stretch. Remain for two to three breaths. Switch the legs

Leg Stretch

Sit on the chair and extend your legs with your heels on the ground. Place your hands behind your head, keep your elbows out and shoulders rolled back. Look forward.

Hinge from your waist; keep your back straight, and lower your upper body as far as possible. Feel the stretch behind your legs.

Keep here for three to five breaths and return to a sitting position.

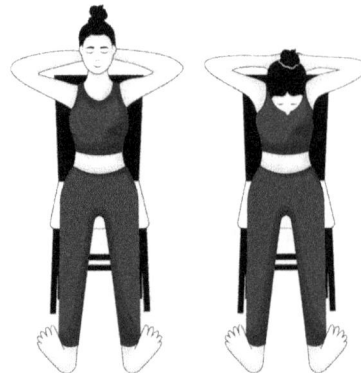

Seated Quad Stretch

Move to the left side of your chair. Keep the right leg on the chair and bring the left foot back. Feel the stretch in your left quad. If you don't feel it, then gently lean back into it. Stay in the position for a few breaths and repeat on the opposite side.

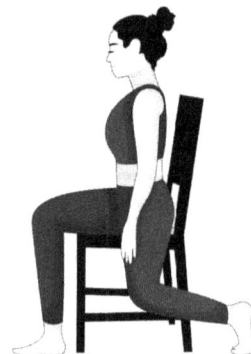

Seated Figure Four or Pigeon Pose

Put your right ankle over the left knee or on the left shin. With your back straight, lean forward and remain for a few breaths, feeling the stretch in your hip. Repeat on the other side.

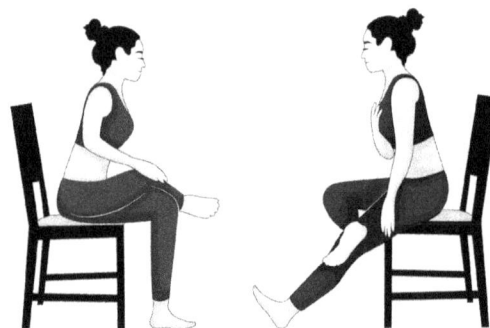

DAY 1

Seated Arm Flow

Bring both arms in front of you with palms touching. Leave left arm in front of you as the right opens parallel to the shoulder-level floor. Move your head to the right. Return the right arm to the middle and repeat to the opposite side—alternate and repeat ten to twelve times.

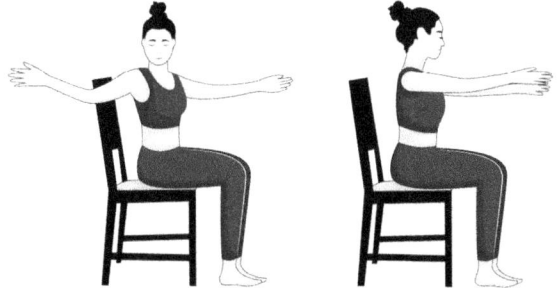

Arm Swings

Allow your arms to swing forward, hands crossing over each other. Swing arms back, then forward again, alternating which hand swings over the top of the other. Continue the movement ten to twelve times.

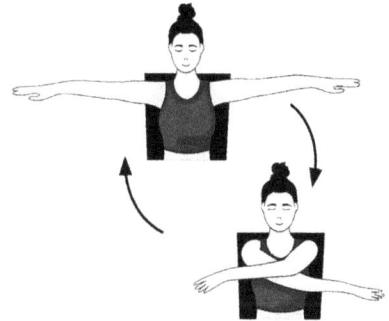

Front Arm Raise

Lift your arms above your head in coordination with lifting your heels. Lower the arms halfway in front of you, at shoulder level, with palms facing each other. Lower the heels simultaneously with the arms. Repeat eight to ten times.

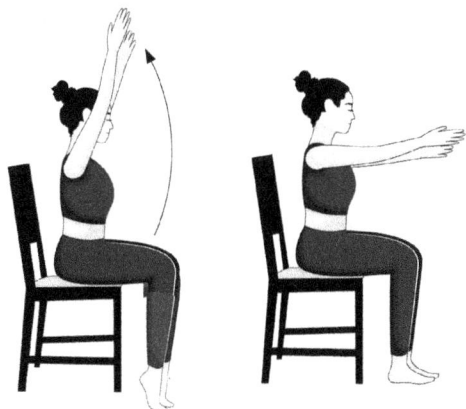

Leg and Arm Lift

Engage your core with the belly button pulled in. Raise both arms and lift one leg and lower. Alternate and repeat twelve to fourteen times.

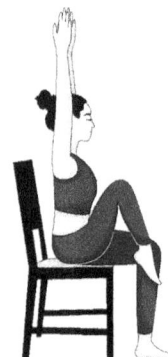

Torso Twist with Straight Arms

Straighten your arms in front of you, join the palms together—alternate twisting to the sides. Repeat ten to twelve times.

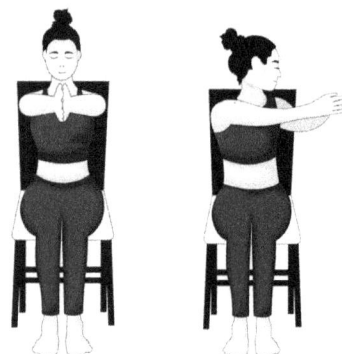

Seated Shoulder Press

You can use weights if you want to, as this depends on your physical abilities. Using your body weight is also great for the workout. Engage the core muscles.

Begin with both elbows extended to the sides under the shoulders, chest lifted. Face forward with palms turned outward. Extend the arms upward, reaching above the head until fully extended or to a comfortable range. Avoid touching the hands together, and keep both arms parallel. Gradually lower the hands to the starting position and maintain spread elbows. Avoid tucking the elbows toward the body's center; extend them outward until a gentle pinching sensation (not painful) is felt at the shoulder blades' top. Repeat eight to ten times.

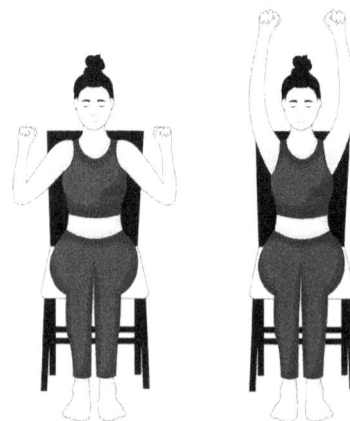

Modified Jumping Jacks

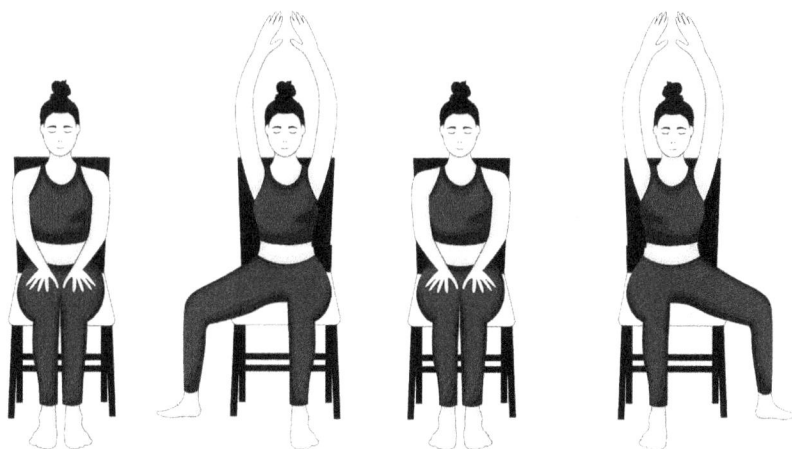

Move closer to the front of the chair with arms at your sides. In a harmonious motion, lift your arms overhead, fingertips gently meeting, with palms turned outward. Simultaneously, extend one leg outward with toes touching the ground as your arms ascend. Bring the extended leg back to the center as you lower your arms. Alternate and repeat eighteen to twenty times.

Skip Rope

Rope skipping—imitate rope skipping using an imaginary rope.

Repeat thirty times.

Your first day is completed. I hope you enjoyed it. Don't forget to do your cooldown routine.

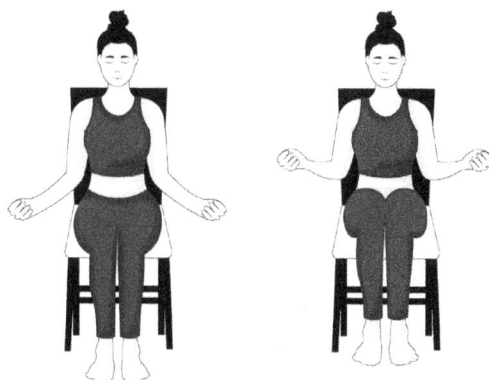

DAY 2

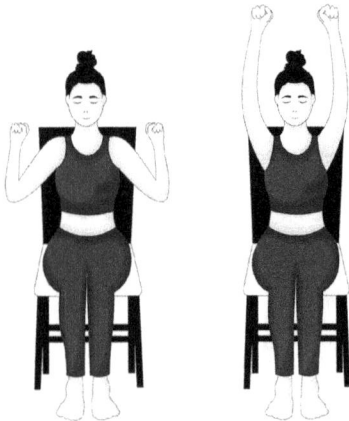

Seated Shoulder Press

You can use weights if you want to, as this depends on your physical abilities. Using your body weight is also great for the workout. Engage the core muscles.

Begin with both elbows extended to the sides under the shoulders, chest lifted. Face forward with palms turned outward. Extend the arms upward, reaching above the head until fully extended or to a comfortable range. Avoid touching the hands together, and keep both arms parallel. Gradually lower the hands to the starting position and maintain spread elbows. Avoid tucking the elbows toward the body's center; extend them outward until a gentle pinching sensation (not painful) is felt at the shoulder blades' top. Repeat eight to ten times.

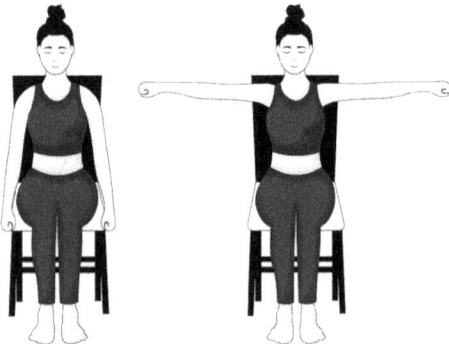

Lateral Arm Raises

Ensure your back is straight. Engage your abs. Place your arms down by your sides. Slowly lift them with weight or without parallel to the ground at shoulder level. Slowly lower them down. Repeat eight to ten times.

Seated Knee Extension

Extend your leg parallel to the floor or at the height that is comfortable for you. Feel your quadriceps muscles working on the front of the thigh. Repeat one leg six to eight times, and then switch the sides.

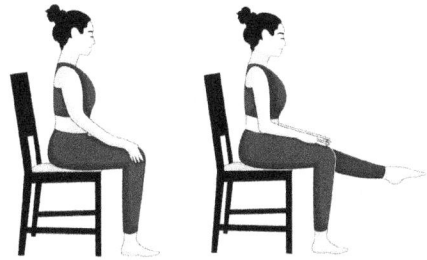

Do two sets for each leg.

Elbow to Knee

Keep feet flat on the floor and shoulders rolled back. Feel your abs engaged. Place your hands behind your head, elbows pointing out to the sides. Lift your right knee toward your chest while simultaneously bringing the left elbow toward your right knee. Return to the starting position with control. Repeat on the opposite side. Alternate and repeat eight to ten times.

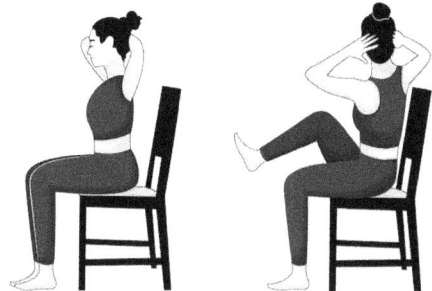

Kick and Clap

Extend one leg forward with a controlled kick, clapping your hands at shoulder height. Focus on utilizing your thigh muscles and ensuring a smooth, deliberate motion. Engage your core and kick with force, maintaining a consistent pace. Alternate legs and repeat the sequence twenty to twenty-four times.

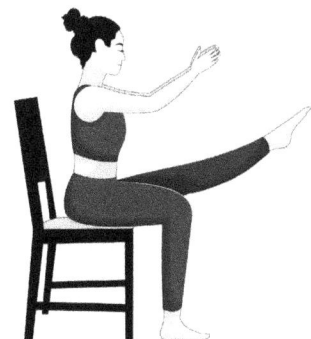

Tap and Reach

Extend one arm diagonally as you stretch the leg on the same side in the opposite direction. Reach your fingertips toward the ceiling, lengthening the arm while stretching the leg. Focus on executing smooth, controlled movements, aiming to create a straight line from your fingertips to your toes. Alternate legs and repeat the sequence twenty to twenty-four times.

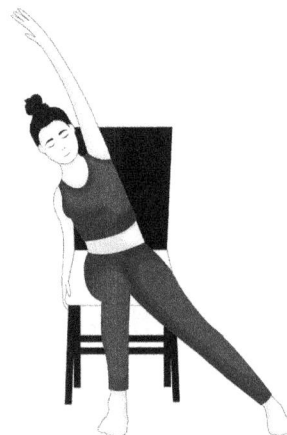

Seated Jacks

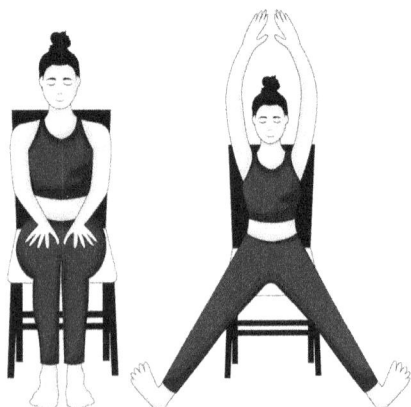

Move closer to the front of the chair with arms at your sides. In a harmonious motion, lift your arms overhead, fingertips gently meeting, with palms turned outward. Simultaneously, extend both legs out as your arms ascend. Bring both legs back to the center as your arms land. Repeat eight to ten times.

If extending both legs and arms simultaneously is too challenging, try this version instead.

Observe your breathing and body. Do it at a pace that suits you.

Try not to hold your breath.

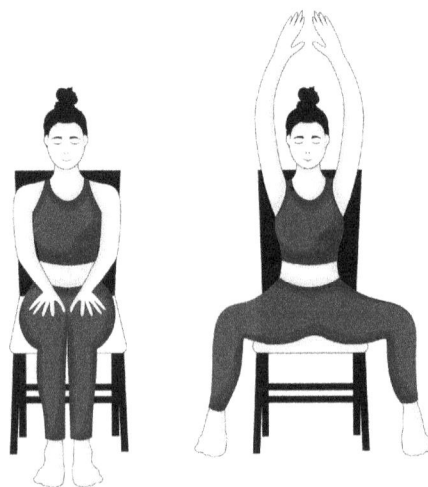

DAY 3

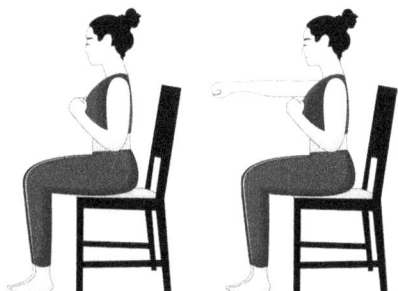

Front Punches

Maintain an upright posture. Engage your core, chest, and arm muscles, ensuring a firm contraction with each swing. Position your lightly clenched fists close to your jawline. With control, slowly punch in front and return to the start position, then switch to the other arm. Alternate and repeat twenty times.

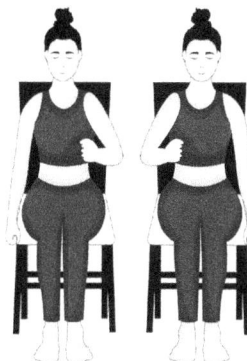

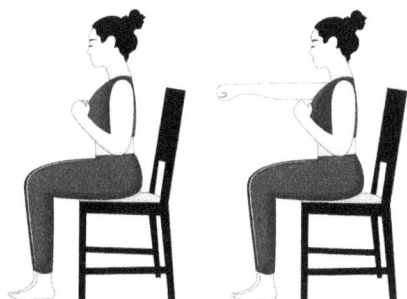

Punch Down

Maintain an upright posture. Engage your core, chest, and arm muscles, ensuring a firm contraction with each swing. Bend your arms and make a fist. With control, slowly punch down and return to the start position, then switch to the other arm. Alternate and repeat twenty times.

Front Punches

Maintain an upright posture. Engage your core, chest, and arm muscles, ensuring a firm contraction with each swing. Position your lightly clenched fists close to your jawline. With control, slowly punch in front and return to the start position, then switch to the other arm. Alternate and repeat twenty times.

Upper Cuts

Sit up with your back straight and keep your feet flat on the floor. Place your hands close to your sides, forming two clenched fists facing you. Bend your elbows, pulling your fists in closer to your body. Punch each fist in an upward motion. Aim to stop the punch around chin level. Minimize unnecessary movement in the upper body. Encourage controlled breathing, exhaling with each punch. As mentioned above, controlled motion to avoid punching yourself in the face. (Real story and experience.)

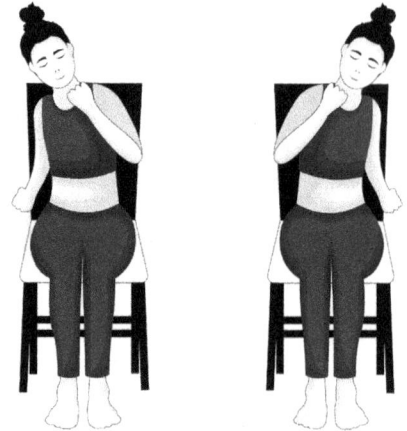

Alternate between your right and left hand for each punch—repeat twenty times.

Start with a slow and controlled pace, then gradually increase speed as comfortable.

Overhead Punches

With control, slowly punch above your head with one arm. Return to the start position, then switch to the other arm. Alternate and repeat twenty times on each side.

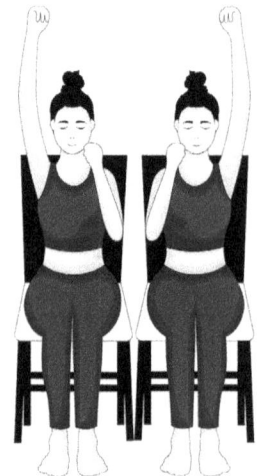

DAY 4

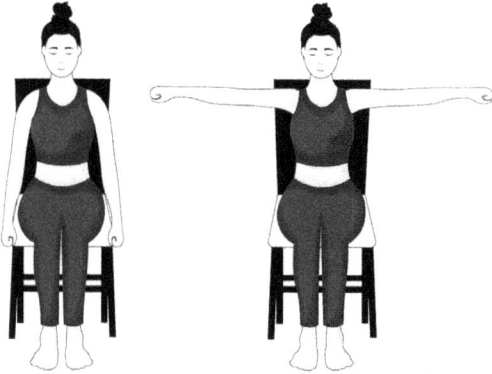

Lateral Arm Raises

Ensure your back is straight. Engage your abs. Place your arms down by your sides. Slowly lift them with weight or without parallel to the ground at shoulder level. Slowly lower them down. Repeat eight to ten times.

Hinge and Cross

Sit straight with knees bent and heels lifted. Squeeze the inner thighs together for more muscular activation. Place hands behind the head and engage your core. Lean back until the shoulder blades lightly touch the back of the chair. Bring your body forward, crossing your right elbow to the outside of your left knee. Return to start. Repeat for twenty alternating reps.

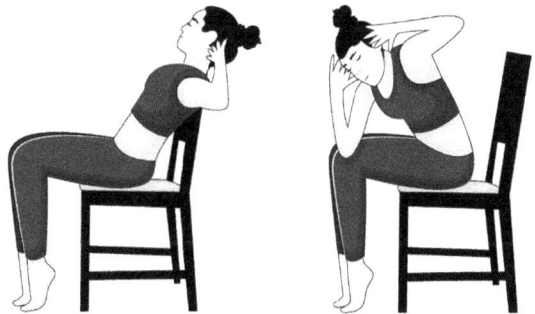

Extended Leg Raises

Engage your abs and lean back about 45 degrees. Feel your abs tighten.

Grab the sides of the chair if you need to. Stretch both legs in front of you and lift one leg. Feel your lower abdominals working. Lower it down and then lift the opposite leg. Alternate and repeat sixteen to twenty times.

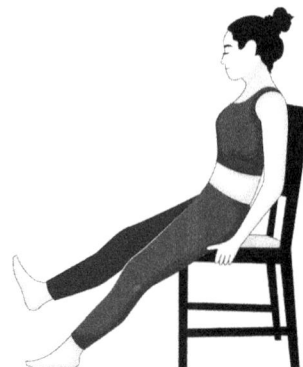

Seated Side Step Over

Lift your right knee and step over the imaginary object on the floor. Lift the leg and step over it. Bring it back by stepping over back. Repeat for eight to twelve repetitions before switching to the opposite leg.

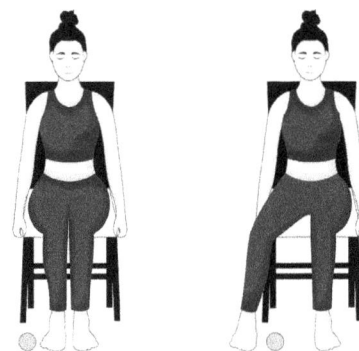

Tap and Reach

Extend one arm diagonally as you stretch the leg on the same side in the opposite direction. Reach your fingertips toward the ceiling, lengthening the arm while stretching the leg. Focus on executing smooth, controlled movements, aiming to create a straight line from your fingertips to your toes. Alternate legs and repeat the sequence twenty to twenty-four times.

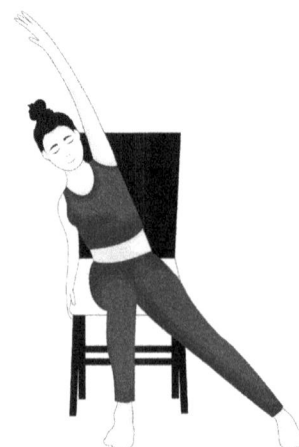

Chair Squat

Start with your knees shoulder-width apart. Lean forward and lift your hips off the chair. If needed, you can hold the chair's edges for support as you safely return to the seated position. Alternatively, place your arms on your knees, but avoid leaning into them. Engage your glutes and hamstrings to assist in lifting your hips. Repeat this movement ten times.

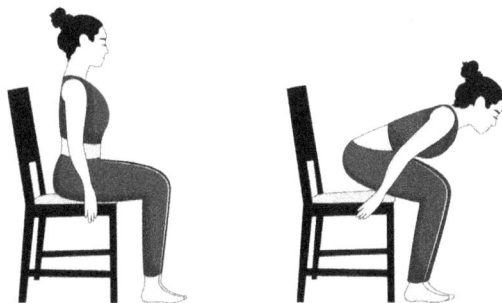

DAY 5

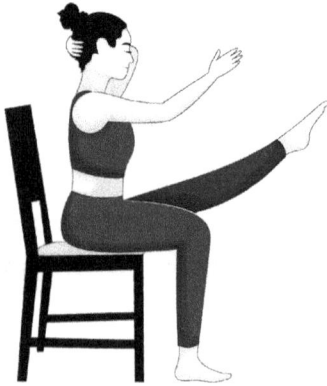

Kick and Toe Touch

Take a short break if you need to. Keep the arms behind your head. Ensure you're not putting all the arm's weight and forcing your neck down. Keep your back straight and core engaged. Arms behind the head. Lift the leg and extend the opposite arm, trying to reach the toes of the opposite leg while the other arm stays behind the head. Alternate and repeat twelve to fourteen times.

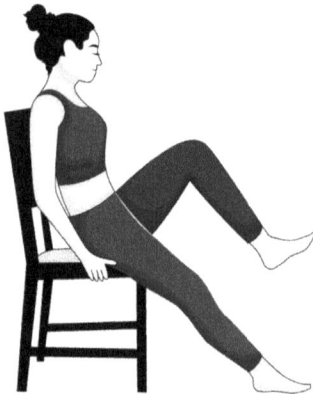

Bicycle Curls

Lean back into the chair and grab the edges of the chair. Extend one leg out and pull the knee back to your chest. Think if you're peddling the bicycle. Repeat on one side six to eight times. Switch to the opposite side. Now reverse—start with one leg peddling in the opposite direction. Switch sides and repeat six to eight times.

Single March with a Twist

Lean back into the chair with your back straight; don't round your back. Move the bottom

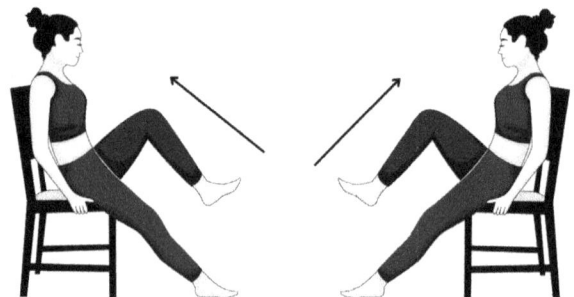

toward the edge of the chair. You can hold the edges of the chair with your arms. Core engaged. Do single marches by lifting your knee as high as you can. Alternate and repeat ten to fourteen times.

If you're feeling brave and strong, lift both knees simultaneously. Repeat six to eight times.

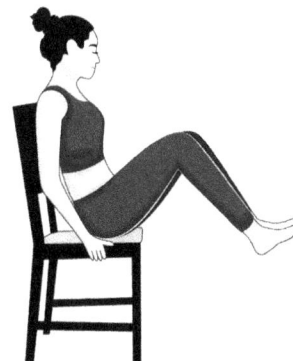

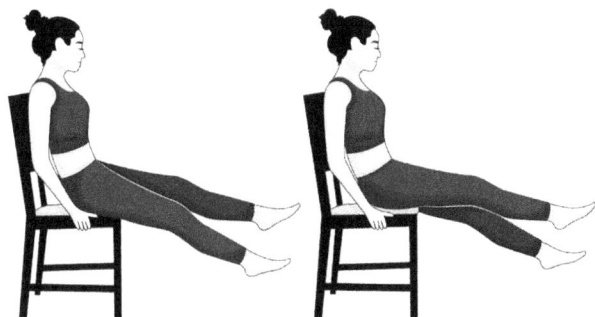

Flutter Kicks

Lean back into the chair with your spine straight. Fully extend your legs, hold the chair's edges, lift both legs, and flutter. Kick your legs up and down. Repeat twenty times.

Chair Pose Above Chair

Maintain an upright posture and lift your arms above your head while exhaling deeply. Inhale and move into a chair pose, gently raising yourself to your feet above the chair. Exhale and return to a seated position, arms still extended overhead. Inhale again and resume the chair pose. Repeat this sequence six times to ten times.

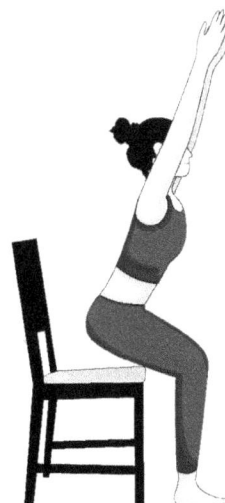

DAY 6

Modify Chair Squat

Start with your knees shoulder-width apart. Lean forward and lift your hips off the chair. If needed, you can hold the chair's edges for support as you safely return to the seated position. Alternatively, place your arms on your knees, but avoid leaning into them. Engage your glutes and hamstrings to assist in lifting your hips. Repeat this movement ten times.

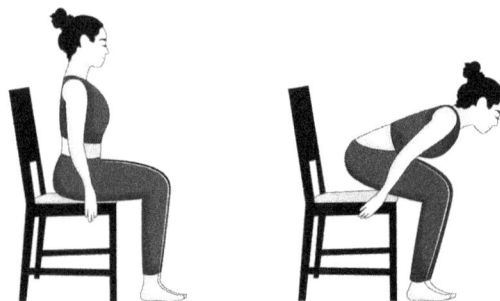

Straight Leg Raise Twist

Position yourself at the front of the chair. Extend your right leg while ensuring your left foot stays grounded. Cross your arms over your chest and engage your abdominal muscles..Rotate your torso to the right, lifting your right leg.

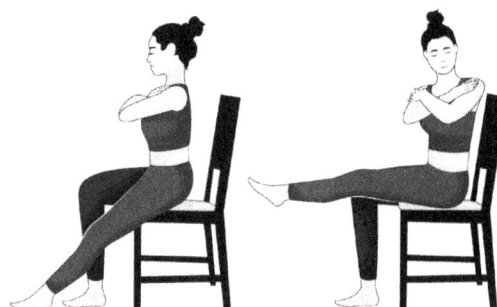

Squeeze your knees together and return to the starting position.

Switch sides and repeat. Alternate and repeat sixteen to twenty repetitions.

Seated Jacks with Straight Arms

Put the palms together with straight arms in front of you. Hold your kneés together. Move closer to the front of the chair if you need to. Open your arms to the sides and step the right foot out to the sides. Open your hips as much as you can. Arms are returning to the middle, the same as the right foot. Alternate and repeat a total of twenty times.

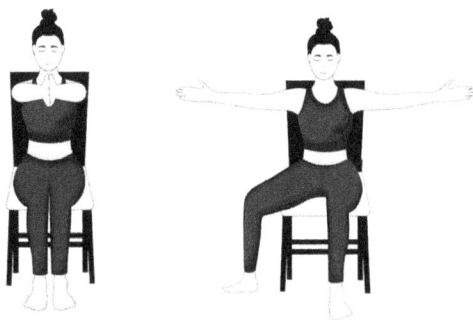

Lateral and Front Arm Raises

Ensure your back is straight. Engage your abs. Place your arms down by your sides. Slowly lift them with weight or without parallel to the ground at shoulder level. Slowly lower them down. Lift them in front of you—shoulder level and lower them down. Control the movement; don't swing your arms. Repeat eight to ten times. You can add weights.

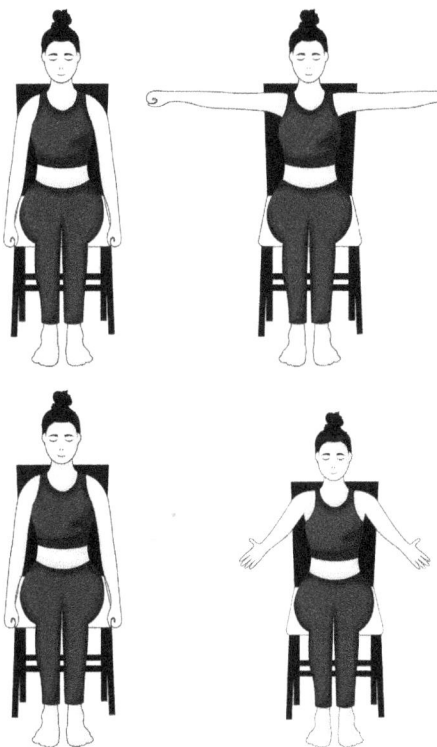

Seat Hollow body

Come to the front of the chair, and with your back straight, raise your arms. Lean back at about a 45-degree angle. You should feel a contraction in your abdominals. If it feels too much with your hands over your head, cross the arms on your chest and hold. Focus on your abs. Maintain the back straight and keep leaning back.

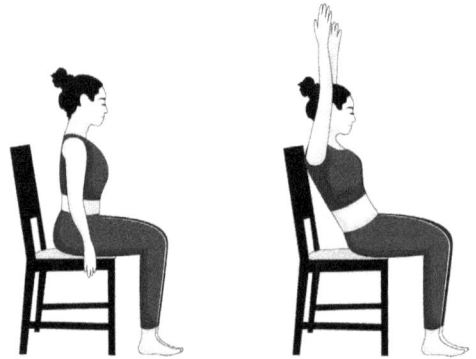

Slowly count to 30. Take a few breaths, rest, and repeat it.

Elbow to Knee

Keep feet flat on the floor and shoulders rolled back. Feel your abs engaged. Place your hands behind your head, elbows pointing out to the sides. Lift your right knee toward your chest while simultaneously bringing the left elbow toward your right knee. Return to the starting position with control. Repeat on the opposite side. Alternate and repeat eight to ten times.

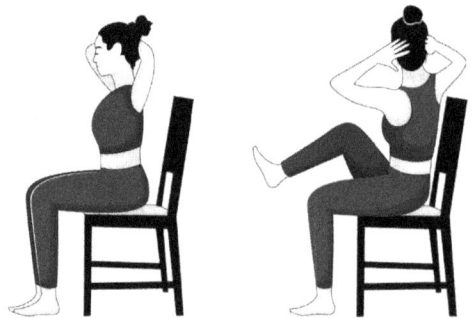

DAY 7

Chair Mountain Climbers Variation

Lean back at a 45-degree angle. Brace yourself on the chair and bring your bottom right to the very front of it. Extend your legs out and get one knee to the chest as best as you possibly can. Maintain a 45-degree position with your upper body. Don't turn this into a crunch. Keep your torso straight, and only your knees are coming toward your chest. Alternate and repeat twenty times.

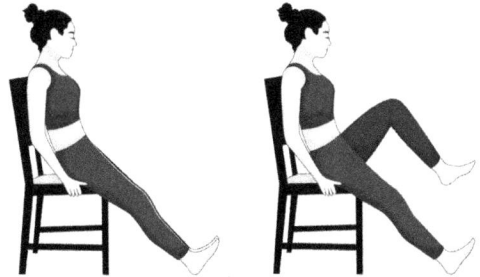

Side Raise and Knee Raise

Keep both legs on the floor with knees bent at a 90-degree angle. Bend your elbows and lift them parallel to the floor at shoulder height. Simultaneously, lift one knee up. Bring the elbows and the knee back down. Repeat with the opposite knee—lift the elbows up with the opposite knee. Alternate and repeat twenty times. You can use weights for this movement.

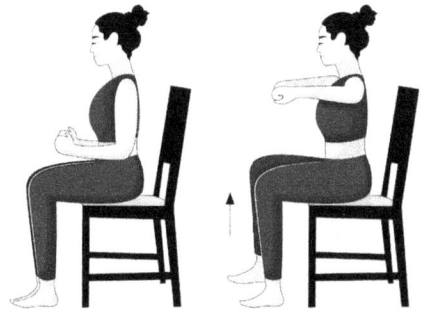

Upper-Body Twist

Engage your core. Keep the chin slightly tucked in. Cross your arms on your chest and twist to the right. Return to the center and then twist to the left. Alternate and repeat eight to ten times.

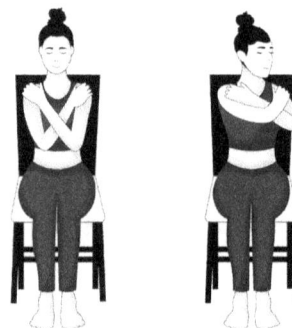

Sumo Chair Get Up

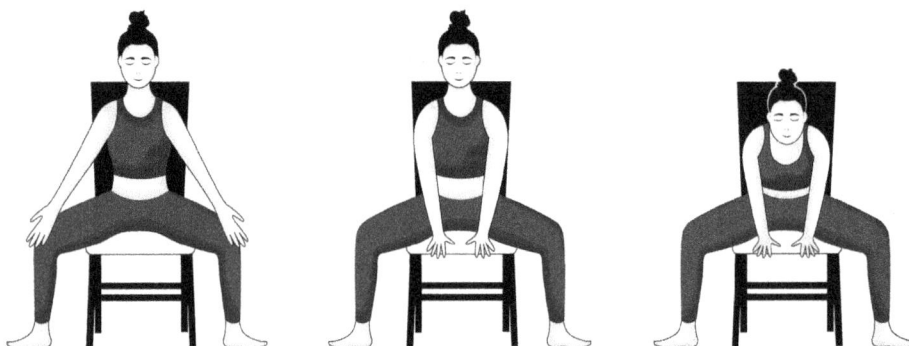

The feet are wider than the hips, and the toes point out slightly. Place your arms in front of you on the chair, lean slightly forward, and lift yourself, but don't fully stand up. Feel your feet firmly on the floor. Don't place the weight onto your hands—the thigh muscles are holding the weight. If you want to make it harder, remove the hands from the chair. Thighs are parallel to the floor. Repeat ten times.

Triceps Extensions

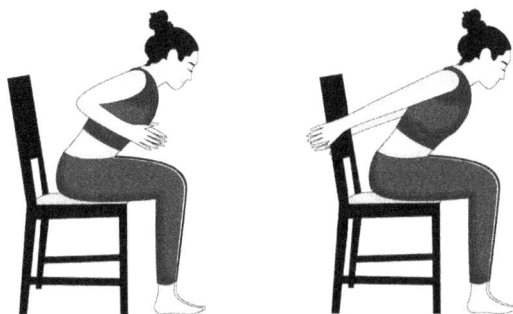

Lean forward at 45 degrees with the spine straight. Bend the elbows and pull them slightly back. Extend your arm back from your elbow; think you are flexing at the elbow joint. If you're working out with weights (bottles or soup cans) that feel too much, drop them and carry on with the movement with no weights. Repeat fourteen to sixteen times.

Seat Hollow Body

Come to the front of the chair, and with your back straight, raise your arms. Lean back at about a 45-degree angle. You should feel a contraction in your abdominals. If it feels too much with your hands over your head, cross the arms on your chest and hold. Focus on your abs. Maintain the back straight and keep leaning back.

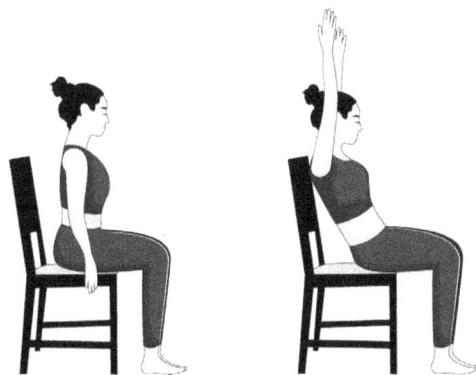

Slowly count to 30. Take a few breaths, rest, and repeat it.

DAY 8

Front Kick and Punch

Maintain an upright posture. Engage your core. Keep your feet shoulder-width apart. Position your lightly clenched fists close to your jawline. With control, slowly punch in front of, up, and across your body with one arm while slightly rotating your torso in the same direction. Simultaneously, kick the opposite leg out. Alternate and repeat twenty times. You can use weights to increase the punch intensity if you need to.

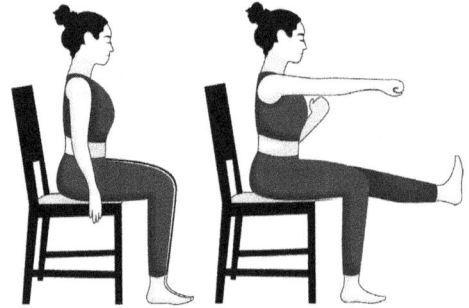

Chair Squat

Start with your knees shoulder-width apart. Lean forward and lift your hips off the chair. If needed, you can hold the chair's edges for support as you safely return to the seated position. Alternatively, place your arms on your knees, but avoid leaning into them. Engage your glutes and hamstrings to assist in lifting your hips. Repeat this movement ten times.

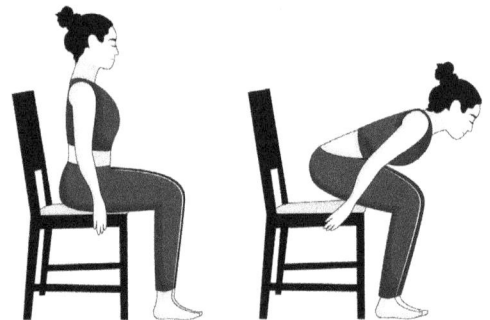

Leg and Arm Lift

Bend your arms and keep them close to your body. It's similar to a marching move. Instead of alternating, you work the same leg. The arm goes up, and the opposite knee goes toward your chest. Lift your left knee with the right arm. Repeat ten times for each leg.

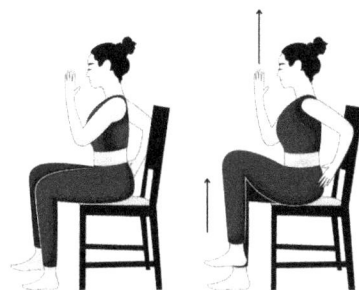

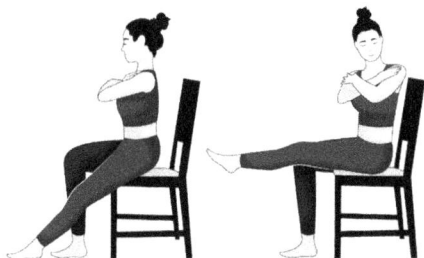

Straight Leg Raise Twist

Position yourself at the front of the chair.

Extend your right leg while ensuring your left foot stays grounded.

Cross your arms over your chest and engage your abdominal muscles.

Rotate your torso to the right, lifting your right leg.

Squeeze your knees together and return to the starting position. Switch sides and repeat. Alternate and repeat sixteen to twenty repetitions.

Hot Feet and Bicep Curl

Sit with your knees slightly apart and elbows next to your body. Start quickly running on the spot—as if the ground would feel hot, lightly tap your soles, and then incorporate a bicep curl.

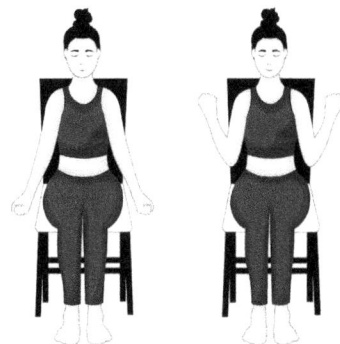

Keep elbows bent at your side, turn your palms up, extend both your arms, and curl. Repeat eight to ten times.

DAY 9

Leg and Arm Lift

Bend your arms and keep them close to your body. It's similar to a marching move. Instead of alternating, you work the same leg. The arm goes up, and the opposite knee goes toward your chest. Lift your left knee with the right arm. Repeat ten times for each leg.

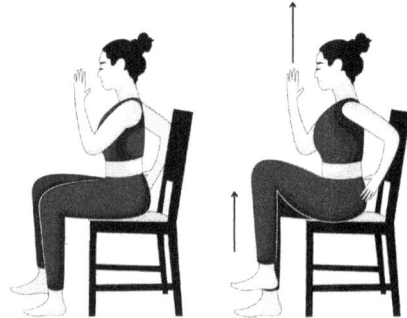

Leg Extension and Arm Crossover

Legs are shoulder-width apart. Arms are straight crossed in front of you, perpendicular to the floor. Extend the heel out simultaneously as you uncross the arms and take them to your sides, parallel to the ground. Take the heel back in and cross your arms. Repeat—uncross the arms, kick the heel out, and bring them back. Alternate the legs and repeat twenty times.

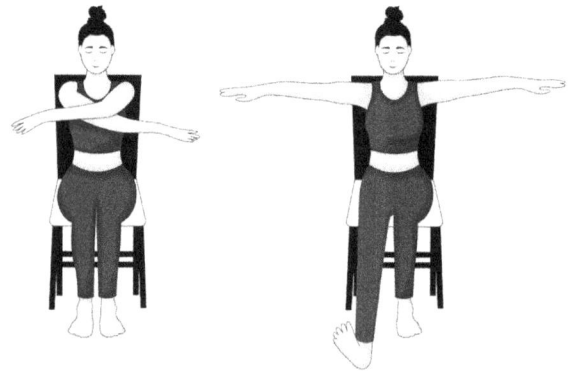

Seesaw Row

Keep your legs hip-width apart. Lean slightly forward with a straight back. The arms are straight and in between your legs. Bend the elbow and pull it back. Lower the arms back. Alternate and repeat twenty times. When you are ready, use weights.

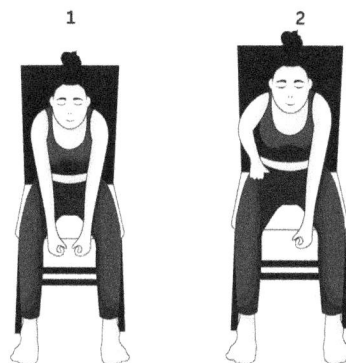

Dumbbell Curl and Kick

Feet hip apart. Kick the right leg out and bring it back. Kick the left leg out and get it back. Hold your arm with a dumbbell with your palm facing upward. If you're not using a weight, imagine that you're holding it up. Slowly curl the weight up (or just your arm) by bending your elbow, keeping your elbow close to your body. Then, slowly lower the weight to the starting position. Now add the kick—curl both arms and right-left kick and keep alternating legs and coordinating with a bicep curl movement. Repeat twenty times.

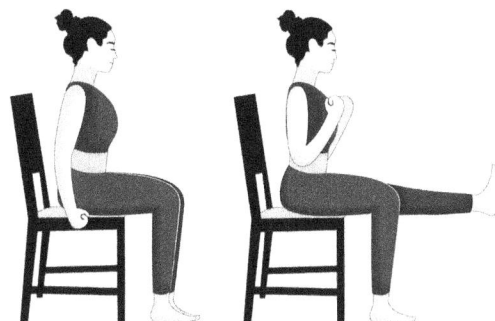

High and Low Pulls

Keep knees hip-width apart. Sit with your back straight. Imagine the rope above your head—extend the right arm up and pull it down. Keep your elbows next to the ribcage. Then, fully extend your left arm and repeat the same move. Both elbows at your ribcage.

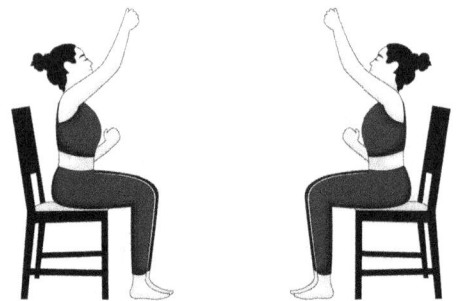

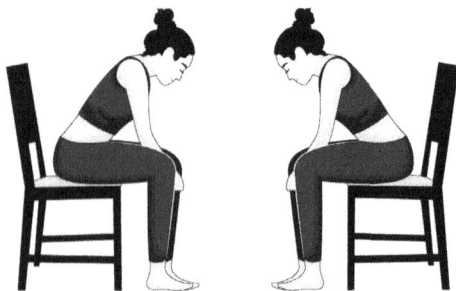

Lean slightly forward and repeat the following movement below your knees as if you are pulling something up from the ground. Utilize both your right and left arms to execute the pulling motion. The sequence consists of four moves: first, pull down with your left and right arms, then pull up with your right arm, followed by your left arm. Repeat this sequence fourteen to eighteen times.

DAY 10

Push and Step to the Side

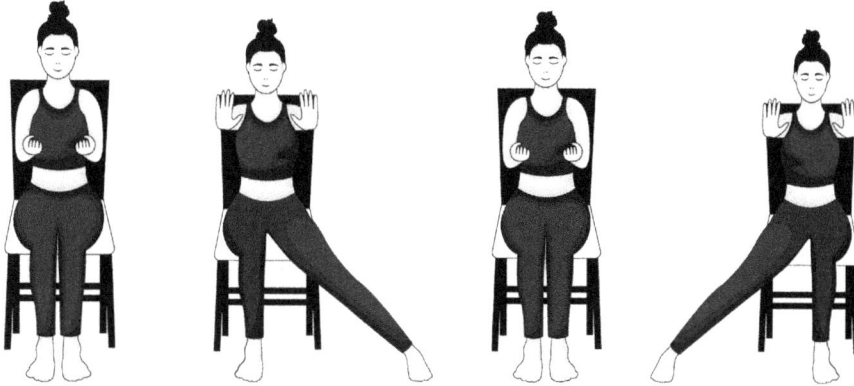

Sit in the middle of the chair, closer to the edge of the seat.

Step the right leg out and, simultaneously, push both arms out in front of you, stretch out, the palms and fingers facing up. Pull your arms back to your sides when the leg returns to the center.

Emphasize the push-out and pull-back arm movement—thirty movements in total.

Torso Twist

Put your arms behind your head and keep your elbows wide. Feel your abdominals engaged, gently twist, return to the center, and turn on another side. Alternate and repeat ten to fourteen times.

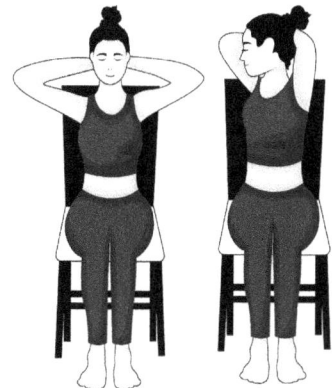

Running on the Spot

Instead of marching, run as fast as you can on the spot for 30 seconds.

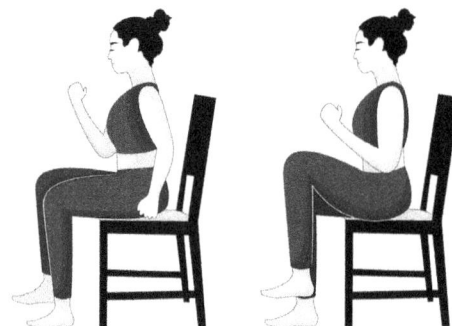

Dumbbell Curl and Kick

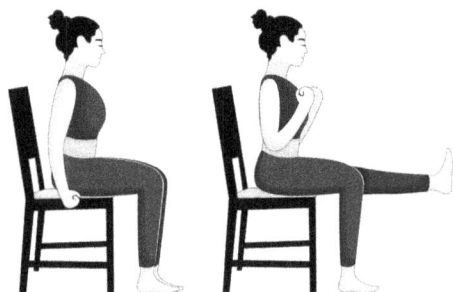

Feet hip apart. Kick the right leg out and bring it back. Kick the left leg out and get it back. Hold your arm with a dumbbell with your palm facing upward. If you're not using a weight, imagine that you're holding it up. Slowly curl the weight up (or just your arm) by bending your elbow, keeping your elbow close to your body. Then, slowly lower the weight to the starting position. Now add the kick—curl both arms and right-left kick and keep alternating legs and coordinating with a bicep curl movement. Repeat twenty times.

Front Punches

Keep your abdominals engaged. Bend your arms up so your wrists are by your shoulders. With control, slowly punch in front of, up, and across your body with one arm while slightly rotating your torso in the same direction. Return to the start position, then switch to the other arm. Alternate and repeat twenty times.

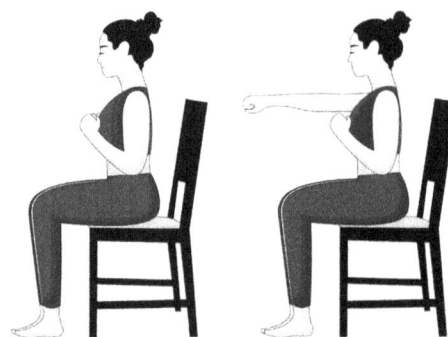

Split Squat Variation

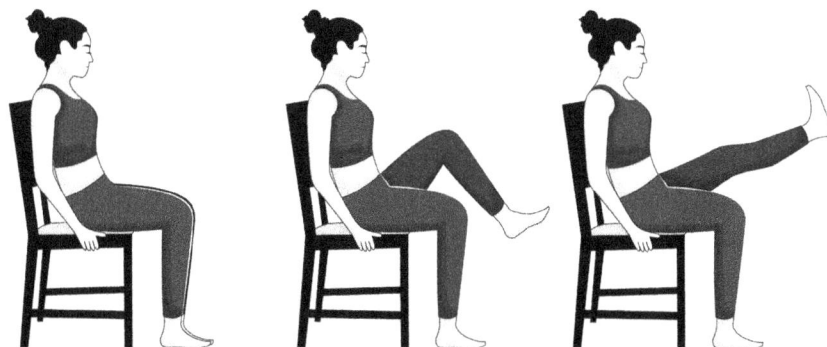

Move closer toward the front of the chair.

Lean back about 45 degrees. If you need to, then hold the edges of the chair. Bring your knee to your chest as close as possible, push it out by straightening it, and bring it back to your chest. Keep repeating this movement for eight to twelve times. Switch the legs, repeat.

Mindfully extend your leg rather than kicking it out. Push it out and bring it in.

Back Bend

Sit nice and tall at the chair's edge with your knees bent. Elbows are bent at 90-degree angles next to your ribcage. Now lean forward from your hips with a straight back, ensuring the head is aligned with your back. Return to the sitting position. Repeat this movement ten to fifteen times. You can hold weights if you can.

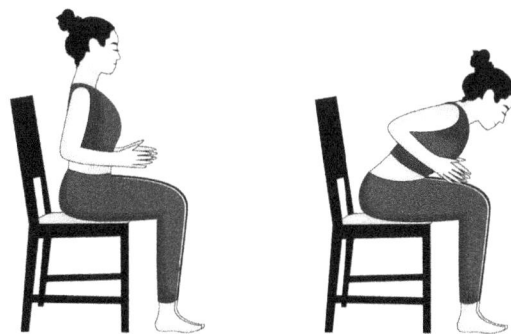

DAY 11

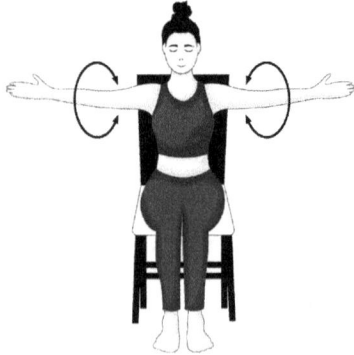

Marching and Arm Circles

Start marching on the spot. Extend your arms to your sides. Keep them parallel to the floor at shoulder height. Slowly start to make small circles and keep increasing them. Complete five to eight moves in one direction and, when reversed, start with big circles, and reduce them back to small circles.

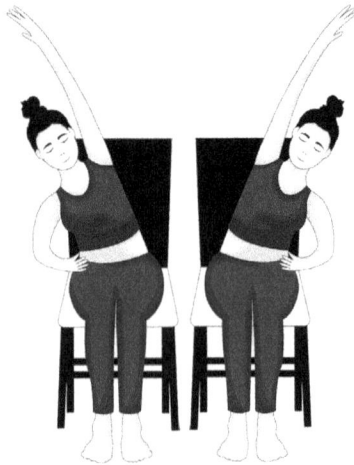

Side Reach

Keep your knees at the shoulder width.

Reach with the right arm up and lean slightly to the left side. Feel the side stretch. Keep alternating and repeat twenty times in total.

Front Reach

Now energetically, keep reaching to the front, slightly angling at the opposite side. Keep alternating and counting a total of twenty moves.

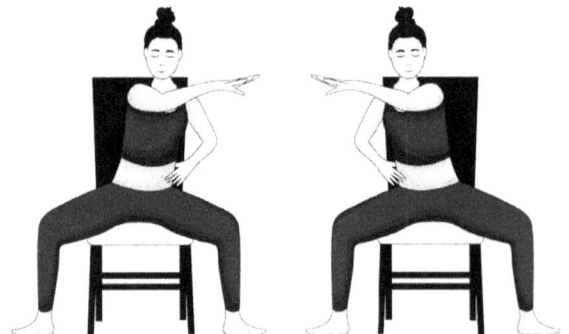

Elbow to Knee

Keep feet flat on the floor and shoulders rolled back. Feel your abs engaged. Place your hands behind your head, elbows pointing out to the sides. Lift your right knee toward your chest while simultaneously bringing the left elbow toward your right knee. Return to the starting position with control. Repeat on the opposite side. Alternate and repeat eight to ten times.

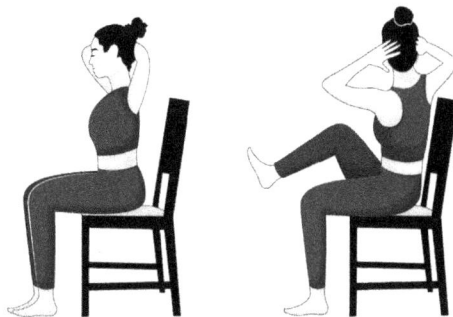

Skater Switch

Shift to the front of your chair.

Bend your right knee while extending your left leg to the opposite side.

Keep your toes pointed.

Start extending your arms. Lean forward and attempt to reach the inside of your right foot with your left arm. Swiftly switch and repeat the movement with the right arm and the left foot. The back is straight. Alternate sides and repeat twenty-five to thirty times.

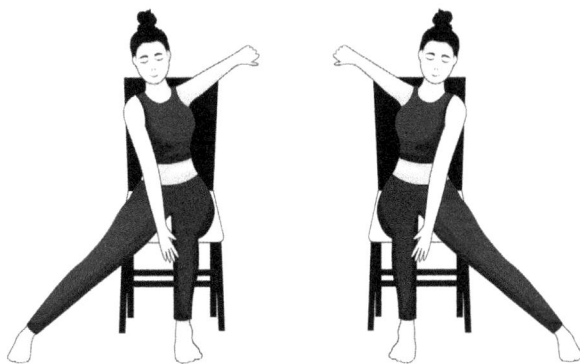

Straight Leg Raise Twist

Position yourself at the front of the chair.

Extend your right leg while ensuring your left foot stays grounded.

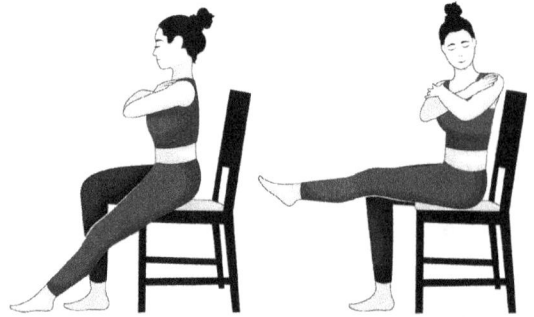

Cross your arms over your chest and engage your abdominal muscles.

Rotate your torso to the right, lifting your right leg.

Squeeze your knees together and return to the starting position.

Switch sides and repeat. Alternate and repeat sixteen to twenty repetitions.

DAY 12

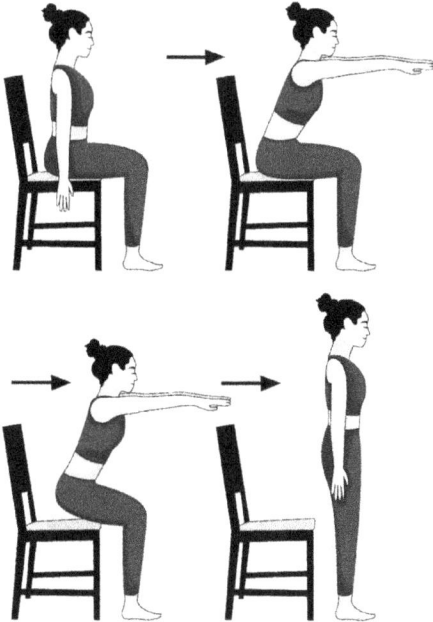

Stand Up Flow

Keep your feet flat on the floor, shoulder-width apart, and underneath your hips. Keep your back and neck straight, with your chest slightly forward. Lean forward and slightly shift your weight to the front of your feet. Slowly stand up. Try not to support any weight with your hands. Take a full breath, and tighten your core and abdominal muscles to control your lowering as much as possible. Lower yourself to the chair with control. Repeat six to ten times.

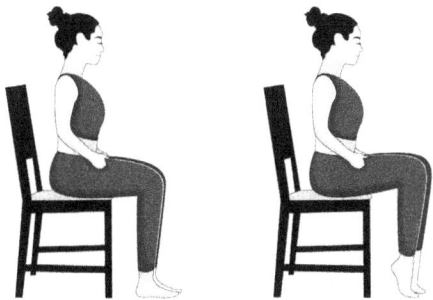

Heel Raises

Sit with your back straight. Ensure that both your feet are straight and the toes are facing forward. The alignment is important.

Lift your heel. Repeat each leg ten times before switching to the opposite side.

Skip Rope

Rope skipping—imitate rope skipping using an imaginary rope.

Repeat thirty times.

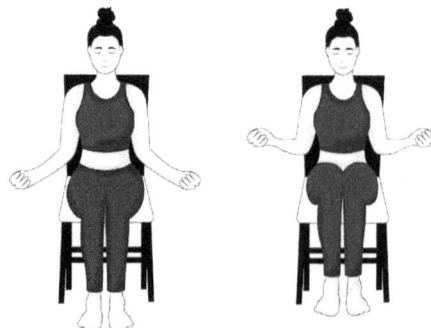

Plank Pose with Chair

Place your hands on the seat of the chair. Stack shoulders over hands, walk your feet back, hip-distance apart. Depending on your body's abilities, walk your feet as far as you feel comfortable. You can be on your toes or feet flat, core engaged. Observe your shoulders being stacked over your wrists. Keep your spine straight. Long line from shoulders to feet. Hold five long, deep breaths or less.

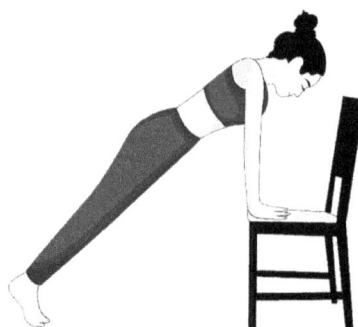

Seated Knee Swirls

Keep your knees together.

Sit in an upright position with your knees together and hold the edges of the chair. Swivel your knees to the side. Keep doing this for eight to ten times.

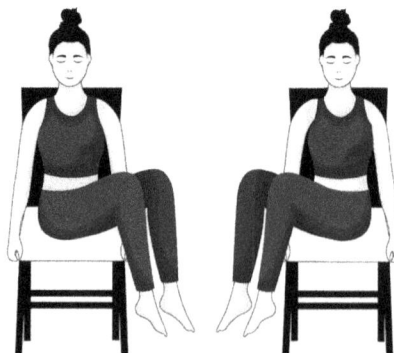

Side-to-Side Punches

Keep knees hip-width apart.

Maintain an upright posture. Engage your core, chest, and arm muscles, ensuring a firm contraction with each swing. Position your lightly clenched fists. With control, slowly punch in front of, up, and across your body with one arm while slightly rotating your torso in the same direction. Return to the start position, then switch to the other arm. Alternate and repeat twenty times.

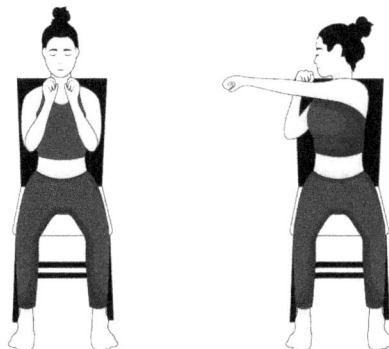

DAY 13

Torso Twist

ut your arms behind your head and keep your elbows wide. Feel your abdominals engaged, gently twist, return to the center, and turn on another side. Alternate and repeat ten to fourteen times.

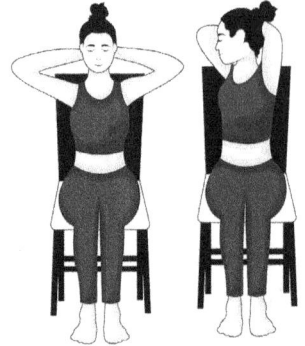

Elbow to Knee

Keep feet flat on the floor and shoulders rolled back. Feel your abs engaged. Place your hands behind your head, elbows pointing out to the sides. Lift your right knee toward your chest while simultaneously bringing the left elbow toward your right knee. Return to the starting position with control. Repeat on the opposite side. Alternate and repeat eight to ten times.

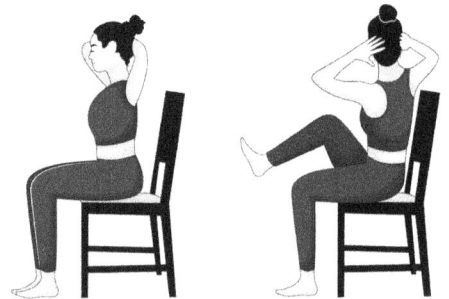

Bicycle Curls

Lean back into the chair and grab the edges of the chair. Extend one leg out and pull the knee back to your chest. Think if you're peddling the bicycle. Repeat on one side six to eight times. Switch to the opposite side. Now reverse—start with one leg peddling in the opposite direction. Switch sides and repeat six to eight times.

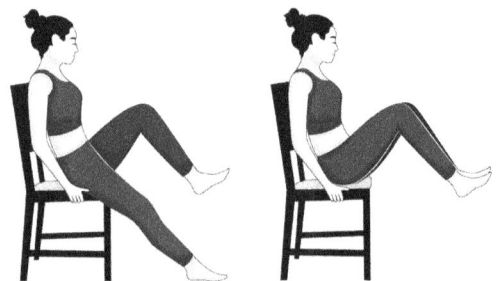

Crossed Arms Crunches

Sit with your back straight and core engaged. Cross the arms on your chest. Now lean back, feel your abs working, and using the abbs, bring yourself back to the straight sit-up position. Repeat eight to ten times.

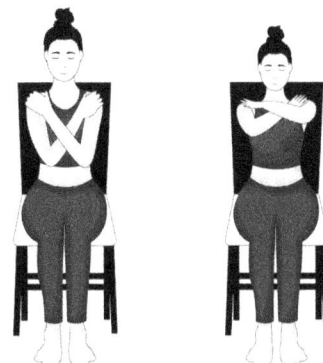

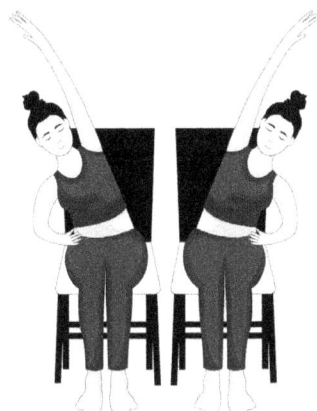

Side Reaches

Sit up straight. Reach the right arm up and reach it over. Feel the stretch and pull yourself back up. Alternate and repeat eight to ten times.

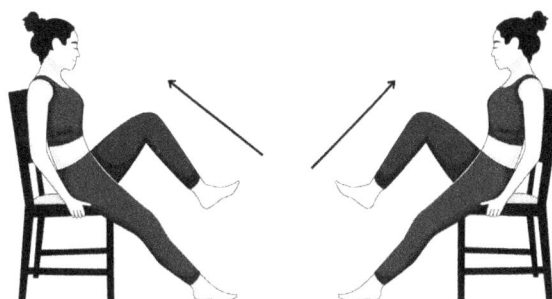

Single March with a Twist

Lean back into the chair with your back straight; don't round your back. Move the bottom toward the edge of the chair. You can hold the edges of the chair with your arms. Core engaged. Do single marches by lifting your knee as high as you can. Alternate and repeat ten to fourteen times.

If you're feeling brave and strong, lift both knees simultaneously. Repeat six to eight times.

DAY 14

Marching on the Spot

March on the spot, counting a total of 50 steps.

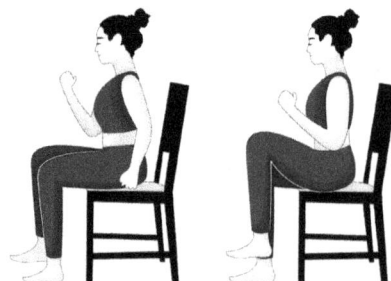

Seated Shoulder Press

You can use weights if you want to, as this depends on your physical abilities. Using your body weight is also great for the workout. Engage the core muscles.

Begin with both elbows extended to the sides under the shoulders, chest lifted. Face forward with palms turned outward. Extend the arms upward, reaching above the head until fully extended or to a comfortable range. Avoid touching the hands together and keep both arms parallel. Gradually lower the hands to the starting position and maintain spread elbows. Avoid tucking the elbows toward the body's center; extend them outward until a gentle pinching sensation (not painful) is felt at the shoulder blades' top. Repeat eight to ten times.

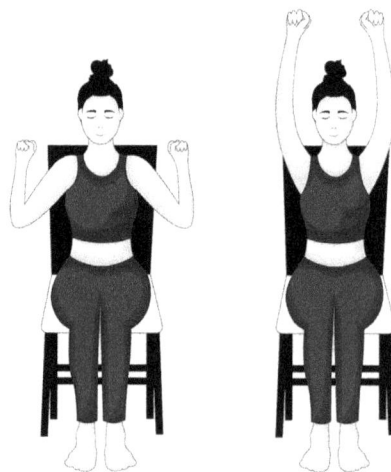

Star Crunch

Sitting on the edge of the seat, bring your arms above your head. Stretch your legs out with heels digging into the ground. Bring your right elbow to meet your left knee and return to the start position. Repeat on the opposite side. Keep your spine straight and repeat alternating fourteen to sixteen times.

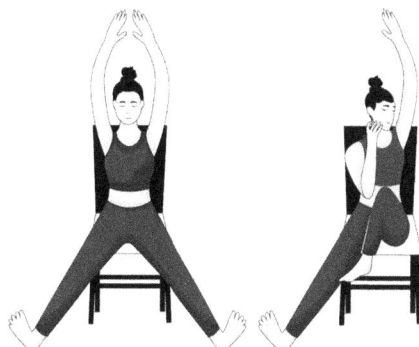

Extended Leg Circles

Sit up straight and lean back into the back of the chair. Kick the leg out (lifted). Pull your leg toward your chest and lean forward to meet your knee. Repeat five to eight times for each leg.

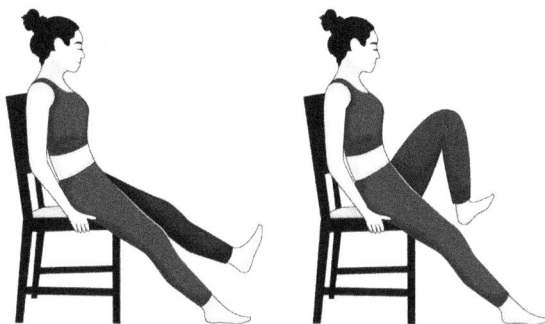

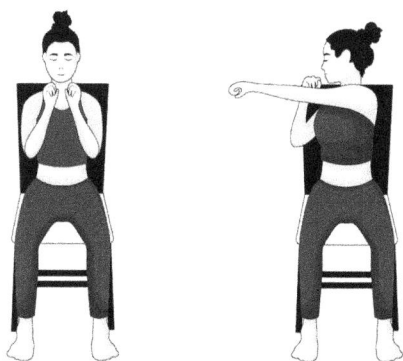

Side-to-Side Punches

Maintain an upright posture. Engage your core, chest, and arm muscles, ensuring a firm contraction with each swing. Position your lightly clenched fists. With control, slowly punch in front of, up, and across your body with one arm while slightly rotating your torso in the same direction. Return to the start position, then switch to the other arm. Alternate and repeat twenty times.

Overhead Punches

Bend your arms, and with control, slowly punch above your head with one arm. Fully straighten it, or as much as you can, and bring it down. Switch to the other arm. Alternate and repeat twenty times.

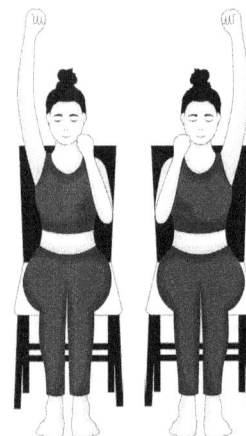

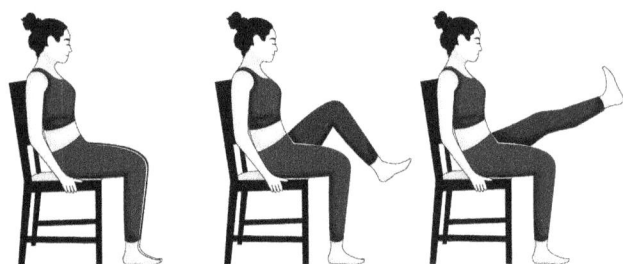

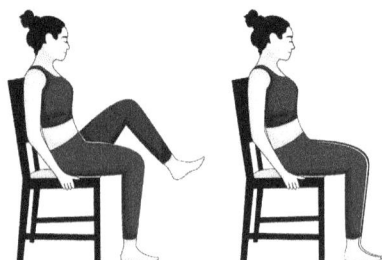

Leg Extensions with a Twist

Lean slightly back and hold the edges of the chair. This is a four-step exercise:

Lift your knee toward your chest, and kick the leg by straightening it out. Then, please bring it back to your chest and lower it on the floor. Work on one leg before switching to the opposite side. Repeat six to eight times.

Sumo Chair Get Up

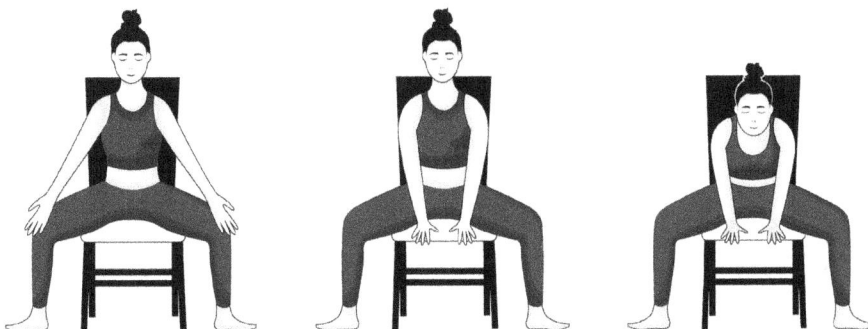

The feet are wider than the hips, and the toes point out slightly. Place your arms in front of you on the chair, lean slightly forward, and lift yourself, but don't fully stand up. Feel your feet firmly on the floor. Don't place the weight onto your hands—the thigh muscles are holding the weight. If you want to make it harder, remove the hands from the chair. Thighs are parallel to the floor. Repeat ten times.

DAY 15

High and Low Pulls

Keep knees hip-width apart. Sit with your back straight. Imagine the rope above your head—extend the right arm up and pull it down. Keep your elbows next to the ribcage. Then, fully extend your left arm and repeat the same move. Both elbows at your ribcage.

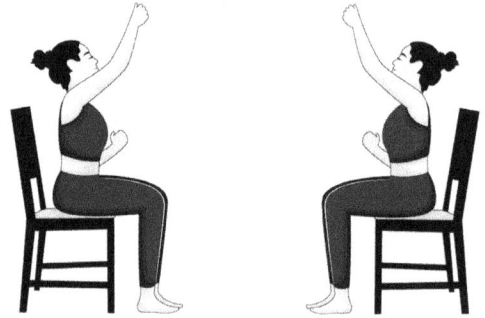

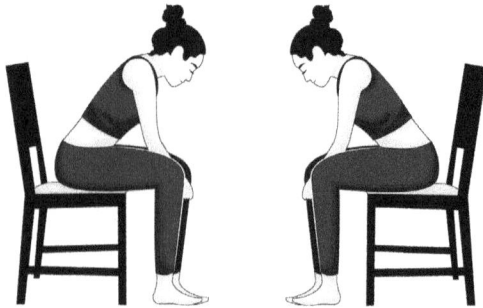

Lean slightly forward and repeat the following movement below your knees as if you are pulling something up from the ground. Utilize both your right and left arms to execute the pulling motion. The sequence consists of four moves: first, pull down with your left and right arms, then pull up with your right arm, followed by your left arm. Repeat this sequence fourteen to eighteen times.

Lateral and Front Arm Raises

Ensure your back is straight. Engage your abs. Place your arms down by your sides. Slowly lift them with weight or without parallel to the ground at shoulder level. Slowly lower them down. Lift them in front of you—shoulder level and lower them down. Control the movement; don't swing your arms. Repeat eight to ten times. You can add weights.

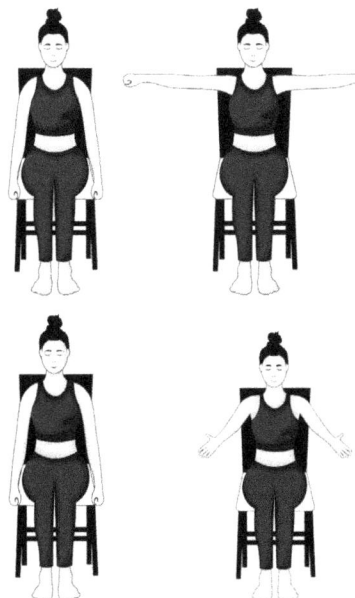

Tap and Reach

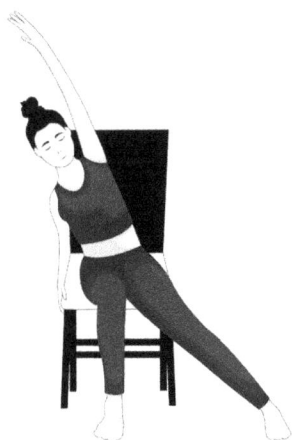

Extend one arm diagonally as you stretch the leg on the same side in the opposite direction. Reach your fingertips toward the ceiling, lengthening the arm while stretching the leg. Focus on executing smooth, controlled movements, aiming to create a straight line from your fingertips to your toes. Alternate legs and repeat the sequence twenty to twenty-four times.

Modify Chair Squat

Start with your knees shoulder-width apart. Lean forward and lift your hips off the chair. If needed, you can hold the chair's edges for support as you safely

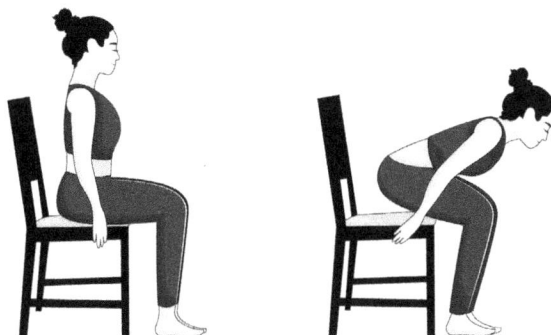

return to the seated position. Alternatively, place your arms on your knees, but avoid leaning into them. Engage your glutes and hamstrings to assist in lifting your hips. Repeat this movement ten times.

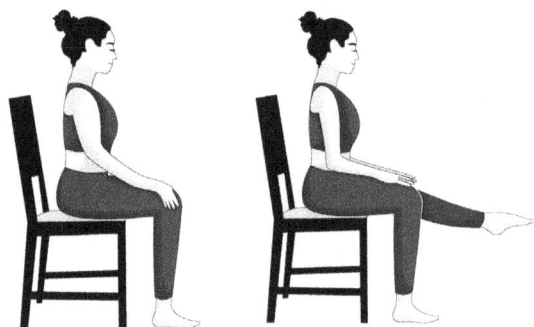

Kick and Toe Touch

Take a short break if you need to. Keep the arms behind your head. Ensure you're not putting all the arm's weight and forcing your neck down. Keep your back straight and core engaged. Arms behind the head. Lift the leg and extend the opposite arm, trying to reach the toes of the opposite leg while the other arm stays behind the head. Alternate and repeat twelve to fourteen times.

DAY 16

Marching on the Spot

March on the spot, counting a total of 50 steps.

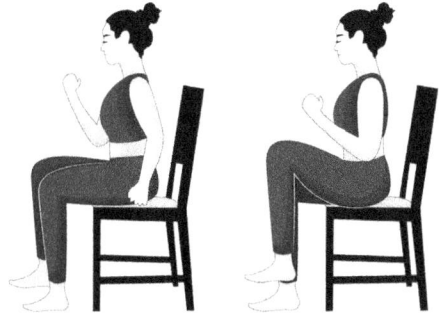

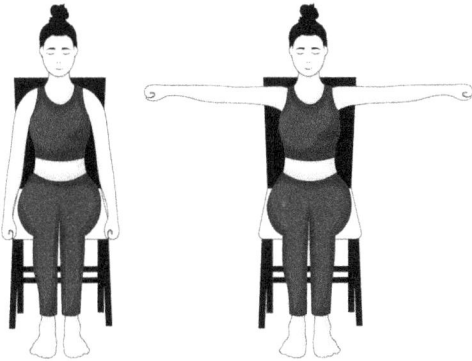

Lateral Arm Raises

Ensure your back is straight. Engage your abs. Place your arms down by your sides. Slowly lift them with weight or without parallel to the ground at shoulder level. Slowly lower them down. Repeat eight to ten times.

Knee Extension

Extend your leg parallel to the floor or at the height that is comfortable for you. Feel your quadriceps muscles working on the front of the thigh. Repeat eight to ten times and then switch the sides.

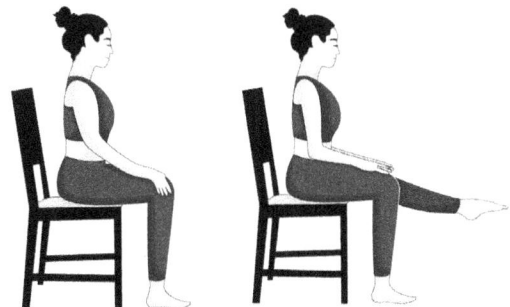

Back Rows

Sit up straight. Bend forward at 45 degrees. Keep your arms straight next to your sides with knuckles facing outward. Raise your arms by sticking your elbows out. Repeat eight to ten times.

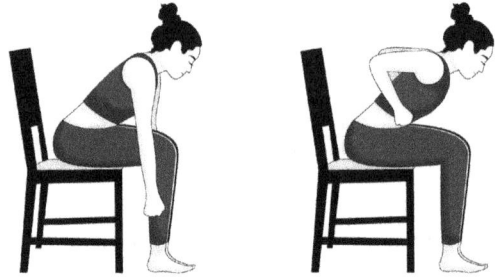

Hip Openers

Sit up straight. Engage your core. Keep your knees together, your arms on your thighs. Open the knees to the sides and return them to the starting point. Repeat sixteen to twenty times.

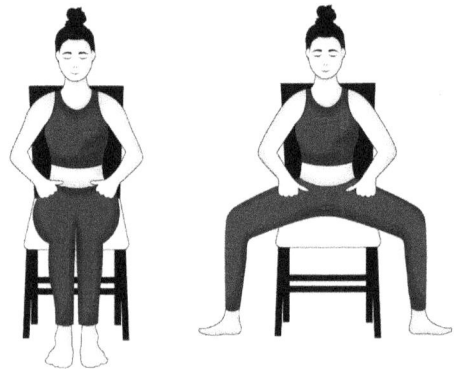

Upright Row

Hold your arms with palms facing toward you at your side. Initiate a gradual lift of the arms, letting elbows lead the movement. Elbows are moving up. Try not to lift the shoulders—only the elbows. Slowly lower it down. Lift your elbows. It's a controlled lift. Lower it down. Repeat eight to twelve times.

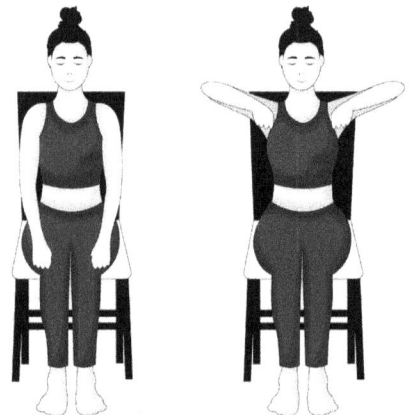

Sumo Chair Get Up

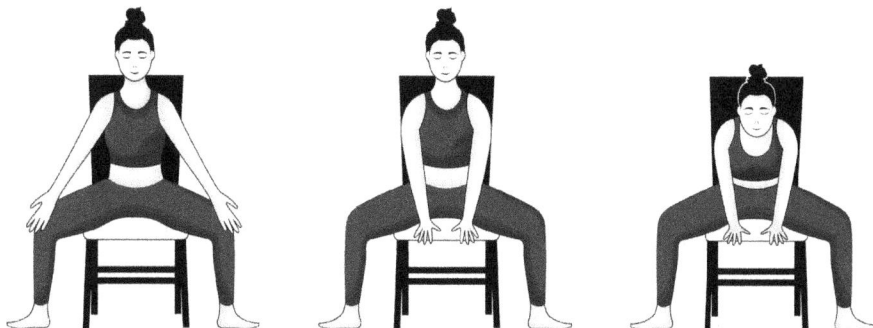

The feet are wider than the hips, and the toes point out slightly. Place your arms in front of you on the chair, lean slightly forward, and lift yourself, but don't fully stand up. Feel your feet firmly on the floor. Don't place the weight onto your hands—the thigh muscles are holding the weight. If you want to make it harder, remove the hands from the chair. Thighs are parallel to the floor. Repeat ten times.

Chair Mountain Climbers Variation

Lean back at a 45-degree angle. Brace yourself on the chair and bring your bottom right to the very front of it. Extend your legs out and get one knee to the chest as best as you possibly can. Maintain a 45-degree position with your upper body. Don't turn this into a crunch. Keep your torso straight, and only your knees are coming toward your chest. Alternate and repeat twenty times.

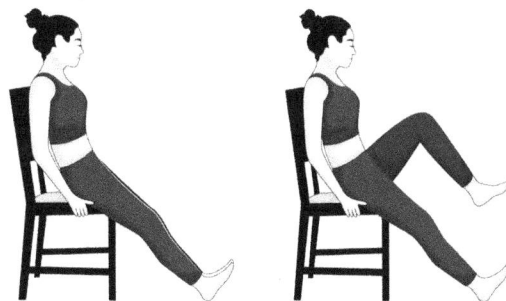

Your sixteenth day is completed. Don't forget to do your cooldown routine.

DAY 17

Front Punches

Maintain an upright posture. Engage your core, chest, and arm muscles, ensuring a firm contraction with each swing. Position your lightly clenched fists close to your jawline. With control, slowly punch in front and return to the start position, then switch to the other arm. Alternate and repeat twenty times.

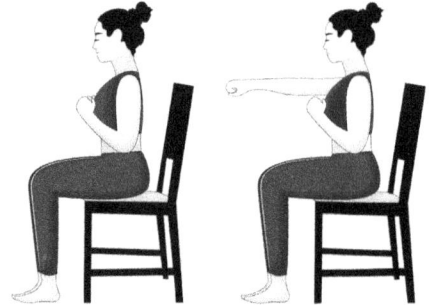

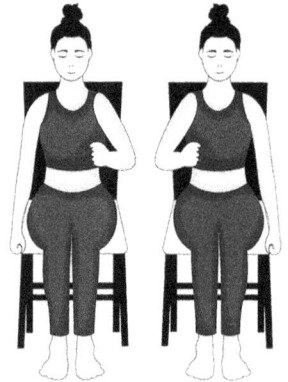

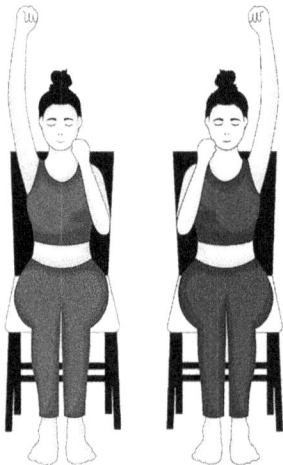

Punch Down

Maintain an upright posture. Engage your core, chest, and arm muscles, ensuring a firm contraction with each swing. Bend your arms and make a fist. With control, slowly punch down and return to the start position, then switch to the other arm. Alternate and repeat twenty times.

Overhead Punches

With control, slowly punch above your head with one arm. Return to the start position, then switch to the other arm. Alternate and repeat twenty times on each side.

Upper Cuts

Sit up with your back straight and keep your feet flat on the floor. Place your hands close to your sides, forming two clenched fists facing you. Bend your elbows, pulling your fists in closer to your body. Punch each fist in an upward motion. Aim to stop the punch around chin level. Minimize unnecessary movement in the upper body. Encourage controlled breathing, exhaling with each punch. As mentioned above, controlled motion to avoid punching yourself in the face. (Real story and experience.)

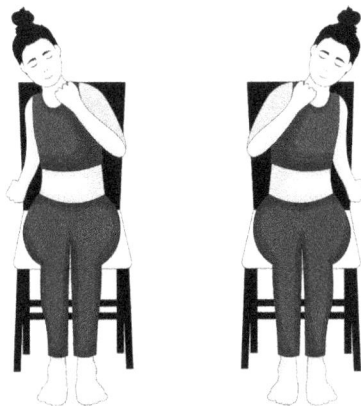

Alternate between your right and left hand for each punch—repeat twenty times.

Start with a slow and controlled pace, then gradually increase speed as comfortable.

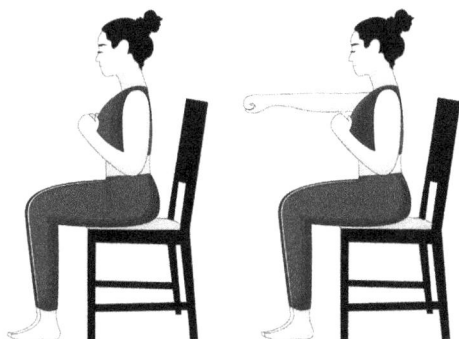

Front Punches

Maintain an upright posture. Engage your core, chest, and arm muscles, ensuring a firm contraction with each swing. Position your lightly clenched fists close to your jawline. With control, slowly punch in front and return to the start position, then switch to the other arm. Alternate and repeat twenty times.

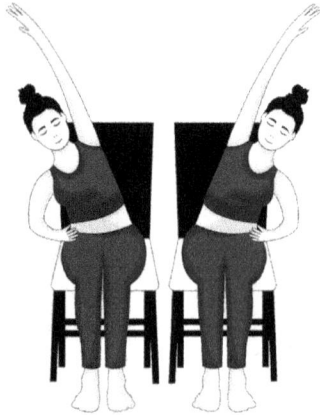

Side Reach

Sit with your back straight and core engaged. Keep both feet flat on the floor. Knees hip-width apart.

Extend the left hand above the head, creating a shape resembling a spoon or a lengthened "C."

Hold the right side of the seat if you need to. Keep your torse engaged; don't let it collapse. Reach with your right arm to the opposite side. Alternate and repeat five to eight times on each side.

Stand Up Flow

Keep your feet flat on the floor, shoulder-width apart, and underneath your hips. Keep your back and neck straight, with your chest slightly forward. Lean forward and slightly shift your weight to the front of your feet. Slowly stand up. Try not to support any weight with your hands. Take a full breath, and tighten your core and abdominal muscles to control your lowering as much as possible. Lower yourself to the chair with control. Repeat six to ten times.

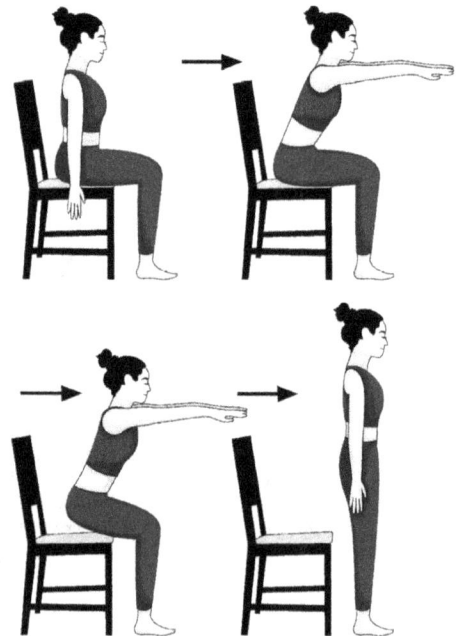

DAY 18

Front Reach

Now energetically, keep reaching to the front, slightly angling at the opposite side. Keep alternating and counting a total of twenty moves.

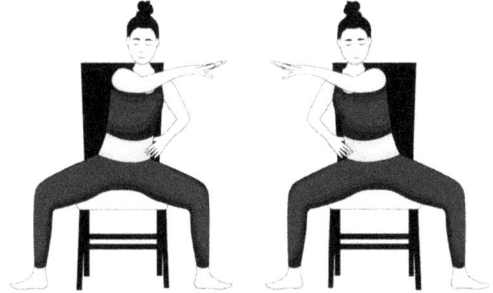

Sumo Chair Get Up

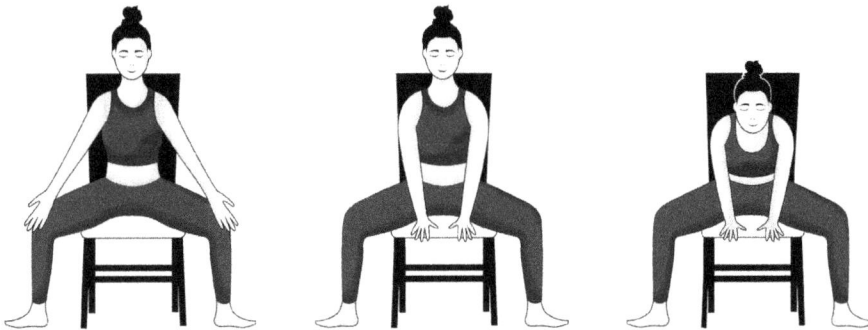

The feet are wider than the hips, and the toes point out slightly. Place your arms in front of you on the chair, lean slightly forward, and lift yourself, but don't fully stand up. Feel your feet firmly on the floor. Don't place the weight onto your hands—the thigh muscles are holding the weight. If you want to make it harder, remove the hands from the chair. Thighs are parallel to the floor. Repeat ten times.

Torso Twist

Put your arms behind your head and keep your elbows wide. Feel your abdominals engaged, gently twist, return to the center, and turn on another side. Alternate and repeat ten to fourteen times.

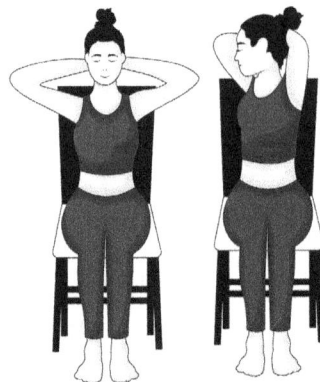

Front Punches

Keep your abdominals engaged. Bend your arms up so your wrists are by your shoulders. With control, slowly punch in front of, up, and across your body with one arm while slightly rotating your torso in the same direction. Return to the start position, then switch to the other arm. Alternate and repeat twenty times.

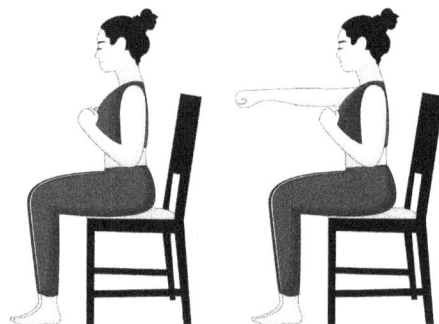

Extended Leg Circles

Sit up straight and lean back into the back of the chair. Kick the leg out (lifted). Pull your leg toward your chest and lean forward to meet your knee. Repeat five to eight times for each leg.

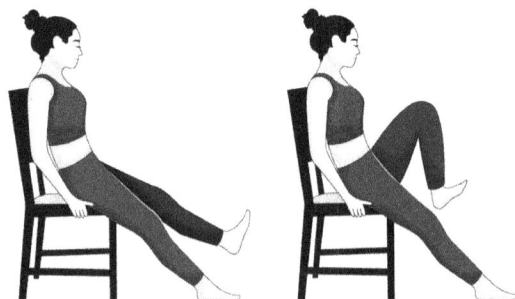

DAY 19

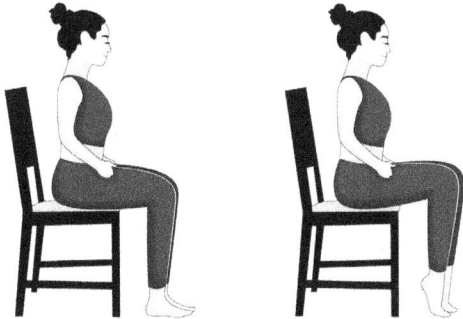

Heel Raises

Sit with your back straight. Ensure that both your feet are straight and the toes are facing forward. The alignment is important.

Lift your heel. Repeat each leg ten times before switching to the opposite side.

Toe Lifts

Sit with your back straight. Ensure that both your feet are straight and the toes are facing forward. The alignment is important.

Lift your toes. Repeat each leg ten times before switching to the opposite side.

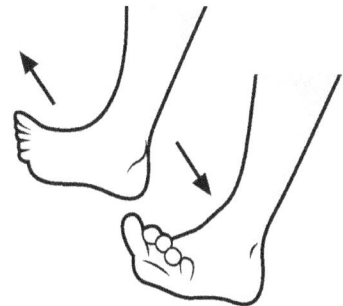

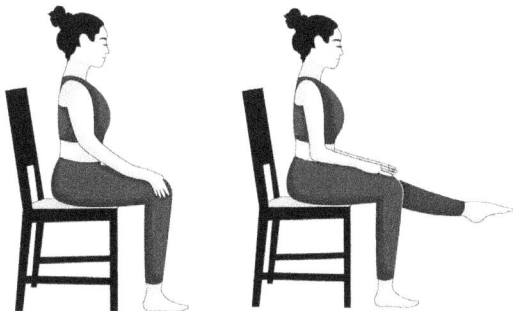

Knee Extension with a Twist

Extend the leg, think of tensing the thigh muscle, release, and lower. Work on the same leg and repeat the movement eight to ten times before switching to the other side.

Stand Up Flow

Keep your feet flat on the floor, shoulder-width apart, and underneath your hips. Keep your back and neck straight, with your chest slightly forward. Lean forward and slightly shift your weight to the front of your feet. Slowly stand up. Try not to support any weight with your hands. Take a full breath, and tighten your core and abdominal muscles to control your lowering as much as possible. Lower yourself to the chair with control. Repeat six to ten times.

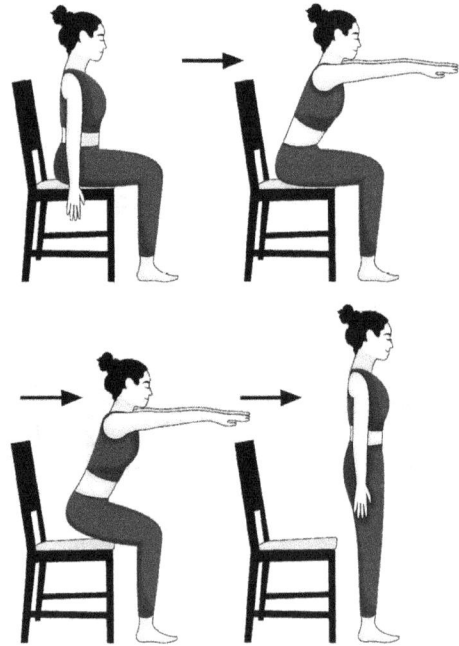

Elbow to Knee

Keep feet flat on the floor and shoulders rolled back. Feel your abs engaged. Place your hands behind your head, elbows pointing out to the sides. Lift your right knee toward your chest while simultaneously bringing the left elbow toward your right knee. Return to the starting position with control. Repeat on the opposite side. Alternate and repeat eight to ten times.

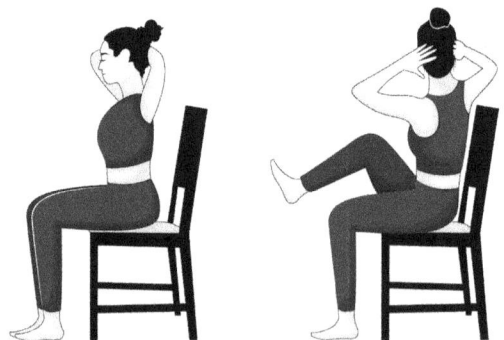

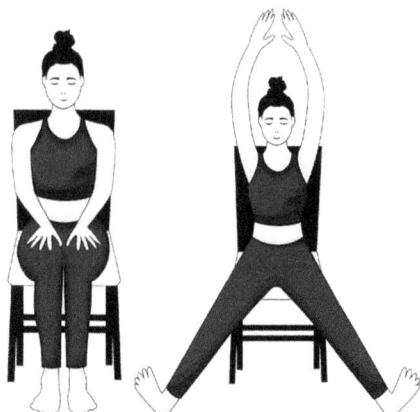

Seated Jacks

Move closer to the front of the chair with arms at your sides. In a harmonious motion, lift your arms overhead, fingertips gently meeting, with palms turned outward. Simultaneously, extend both legs out as your arms ascend. Bring both legs back to the center as your arms land. Repeat eight to ten times.

If extending both legs and arms simultaneously is too challenging, try this version instead.

Observe your breathing and body. Do it at a pace that suits you.

Try not to hold your breath.

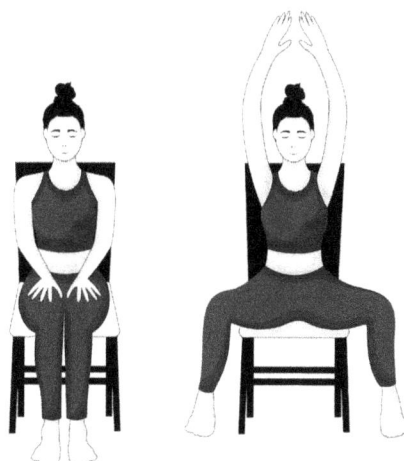

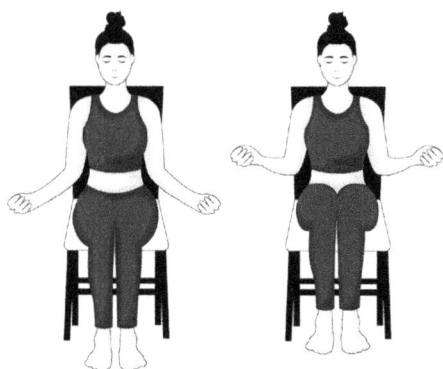

Skip Rope

Rope skipping—imitate rope skipping using an imaginary rope.

Repeat thirty times.

DAY 20

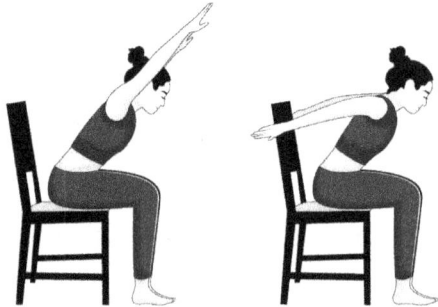

Arms' Push Back

Sit closer to the edge of the chair. Lean 45 degrees forward and lift your arms with palms facing down. Take them back by lowering them and raising them behind your back as if you were making airplane arms. Repeat the movement ten to twelve times.

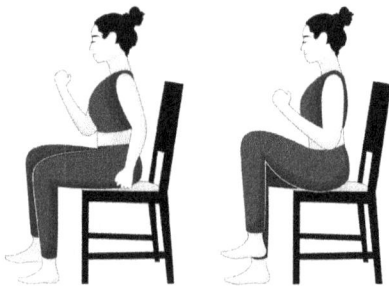

Marching on the Spot

March on the spot, counting a total of 30 steps.

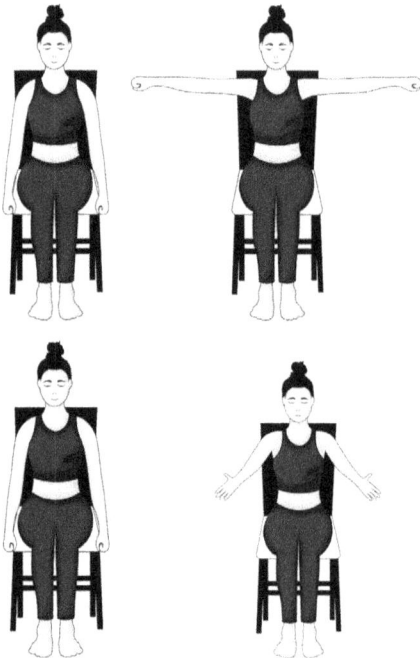

Lateral and Front Arm Raises

Ensure your back is straight. Engage your abs. Place your arms down by your sides. Slowly lift them with weight or without parallel to the ground at shoulder level. Slowly lower them down. Lift them in front of you—shoulder level and lower them down. Control the movement; don't swing your arms. Repeat eight to ten times. You can add weights.

Hot Feet and Bicep Curl

Sit with your knees slightly apart and elbows next to your body. Start quickly running on the spot—as if the ground would feel hot, lightly tap your soles, and then incorporate a bicep curl.

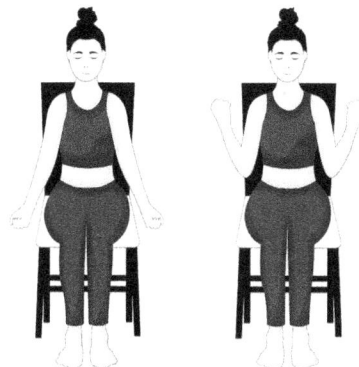

Keep elbows bent at your side, turn your palms up, extend both your arms, and curl. Repeat twelve to fifteen times.

Shoulder Shrugs

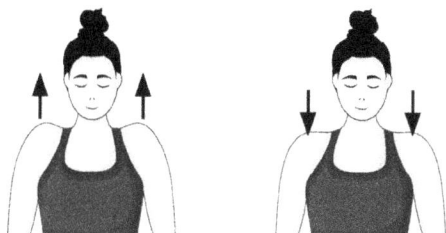

Exhale and raise your shoulders slowly without bending your elbows, as if you're shrugging. At the same time, lift your heels. Keep your hands perpendicular to the floor throughout the exercise. Repeat the process in three sets of eight to twelve repetitions. As your shoulders strengthen with time, you can increase repetitions.

Step and Press

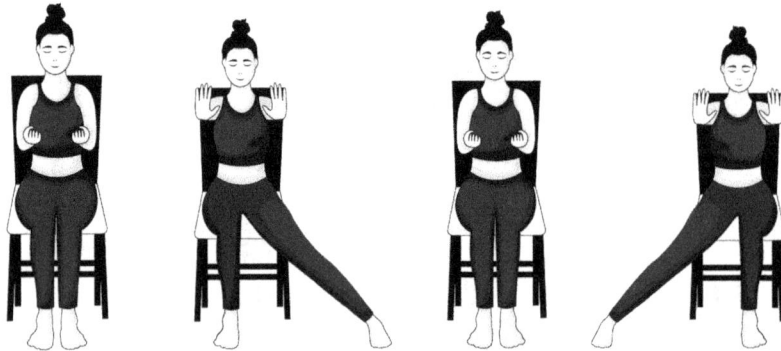

Keep your back straight, and keep the elbows bent with your palm facing out. Make a 90-degree angle on both sides (cactus arms). Press it up, and at the same time, step one foot to the side and keep your knee slightly bent. Pull your arms back and step the leg back to the center. Alternate and repeat twenty times.

Torso Twist

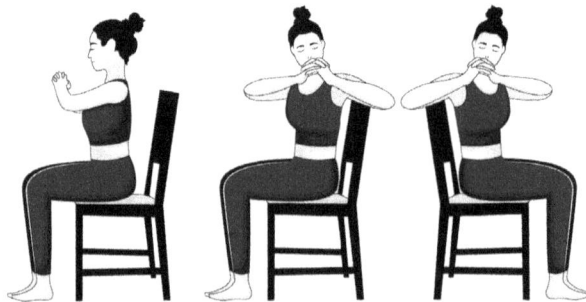

Put your arms in front of your chest. Imagine that you're holding a ball or weight unless you're holding it. Don't press elbows to your sides; leave some space between them. Feel your abdominals engaged, gently twist, return to the center, and turn on another side. Alternate and repeat eighteen to twenty times.

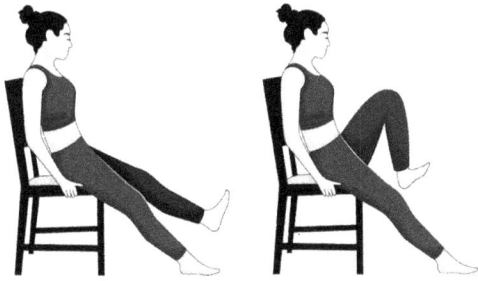

Extended Leg Circles

Sit up straight and lean back into the back of the chair. Kick the leg out (lifted). Pull your leg toward your chest and lean forward to meet your knee. Repeat five to eight times for each leg.

High Knee Pull Down

Put your arms above your head and pull them down, lifting the knee toward your chest. Lift your arms up again, and on the way down, lift an opposite knee. Repeat twenty times in total.

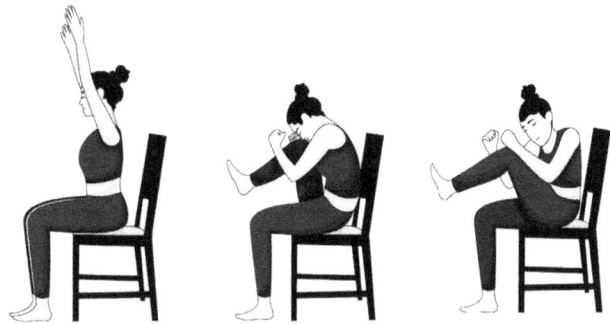

DAY 21

Leg and Arm Lift

Bend your arms and keep them close to your body. It's similar to a marching move. Instead of alternating, you work the same leg. The arm goes up, and the opposite knee goes toward your chest. Lift your left knee with the right arm. Repeat ten times for each leg.

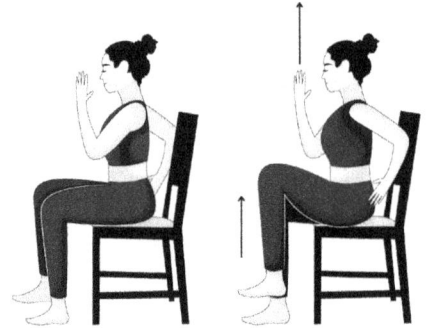

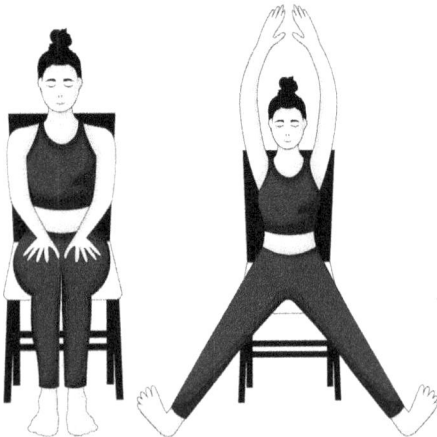

Seated Jacks

Move closer to the front of the chair with arms at your sides. In a harmonious motion, lift your arms overhead, fingertips gently meeting, with palms turned outward. Simultaneously, extend both legs out as your arms ascend. Bring both legs back to the center as your arms land. Repeat eight to ten times.

If extending both legs and arms simultaneously is too challenging, try this version instead.

Observe your breathing and body. Do it at a pace that suits you.

Try not to hold your breath.

Overhead Press with a Twist

Keep the arms next to you with your palms facing in. Pull the elbows up; the shoulders are in line; the neck is nice and tall. Flip the arms over and reach above your head.

Reverse on your way back—pull elbows down (cactus arms), flip the hands over, and lower them to your side. Repeat ten to twelve times. You can use weights if you want.

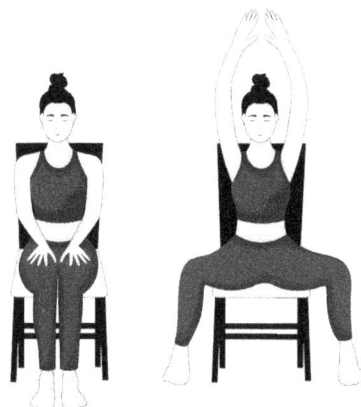

Chair Mountain Climbers Variation

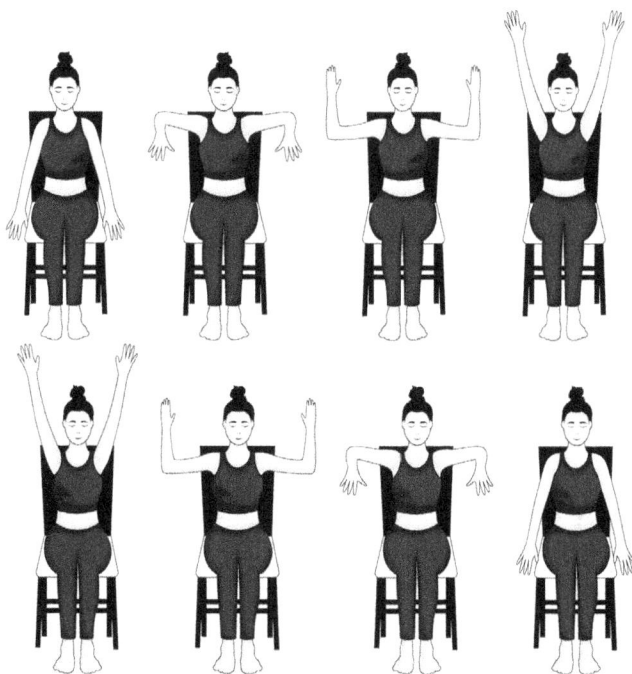

Lean back at a 45-degree angle. Brace yourself on the chair and bring your bottom right to the very front of it. Extend your legs out and get one knee to the chest as best as you possibly can. Maintain a 45-degree position with your upper body. Don't turn this into a crunch. Keep your torso straight, and only your knees are coming toward your chest. Alternate and repeat twenty to twenty-four times.

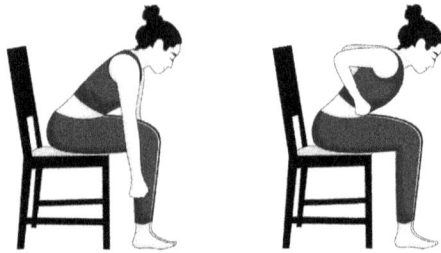

Back Rows

Sit up straight. Bend forward at 45 degree. Keep your arms straight next to your sides with knuckles facing outward. Raise your arms by sticking your elbows out. Repeat eight to ten times.

Step and Press

Keep your back straight, and keep the elbows bent with your palm facing out. Make a 90-degree angle on both sides (cactus arms). Press it up, and at the same time, step one foot to the side and keep your knee slightly bent. Pull your arms back and step the leg back to the center. Alternate and repeat twenty times. You can use weights.

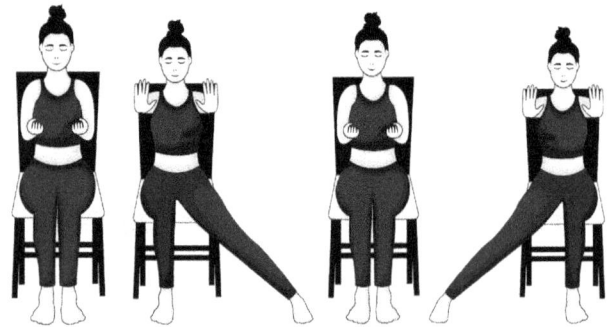

Dumbbell Curl and Kick

Feet hip apart. Kick the right leg out and bring it back. Kick the left leg out and get it back. Hold your arm with a dumbbell with your palm facing upward. If you're not using weight, imagine that you're holding it up. Slowly curl the weight up (or just your arm) by bending your elbow, keeping your elbow close to your body. Then, slowly lower the weight to the starting position. Now add the kick—curl both arms and right-left kick and keep alternating legs and coordinating with a bicep curl movement. Repeat twenty times.

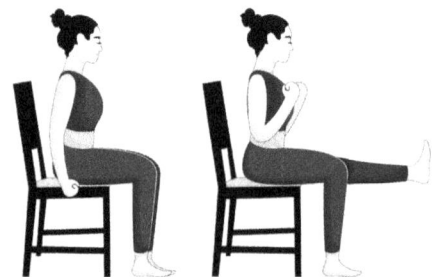

DAY 22

Seated Side Step Over

Lift your right knee and step over the imaginary object on the floor. Lift the leg and step over it. Bring it back by stepping over back. Repeat for eight to twelve repetitions before switching to the opposite leg.

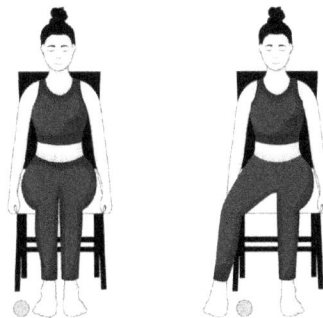

Kick and Clap

Extend one leg forward with a controlled kick, clapping your hands at shoulder height. Focus on utilizing your thigh muscles and ensuring a smooth, deliberate motion. Engage your core and kick with force, maintaining a consistent pace. Alternate legs and repeat the sequence twenty to twenty-four times.

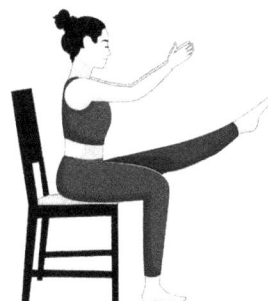

Tap and Reach

Extend one arm diagonally as you stretch the leg on the same side in the opposite direction. Reach your fingertips toward the ceiling, lengthening the arm while stretching the leg. Focus on executing smooth, controlled movements, aiming to create a straight line from your fingertips to your toes. Alternate legs and repeat the sequence twenty to twenty-four times.

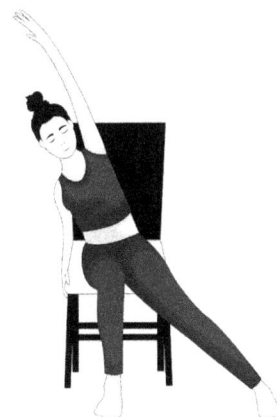

Elbow to Knee

Keep feet flat on the floor and shoulders rolled back. Feel your abs engaged. Place your hands behind your head, elbows pointing out to the sides. Lift your right knee toward your chest while simultaneously bringing the left elbow toward your right knee. Return to the starting position with control. Repeat on the opposite side. Alternate and repeat eight to ten times.

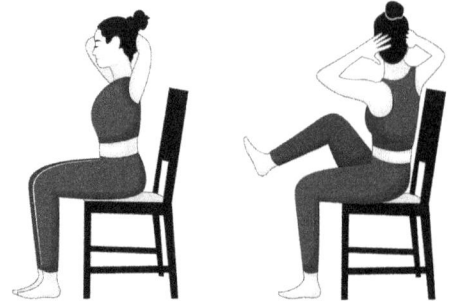

Skip Rope

Rope skipping—imitate rope skipping using an imaginary rope.

Repeat thirty times.

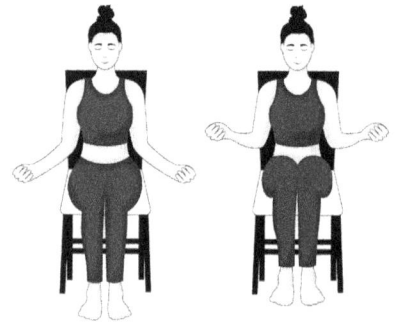

Step and Press

Keep your back straight, and keep the elbows bent with your palm facing out. Make a 90-degree angle on both sides (cactus arms). Press it up, and at the same time, step one foot to the side and keep your knee slightly bent. Pull your arms back and step the leg back to the center. Alternate and repeat twenty times.

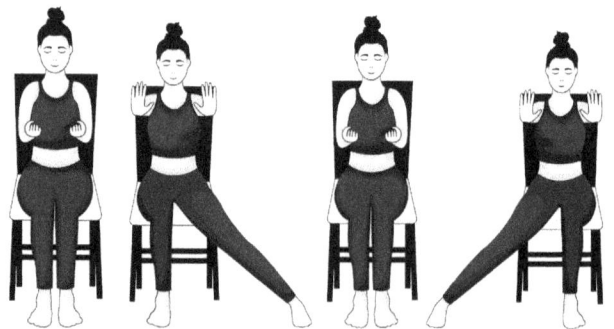

DAY 23

Elegant Kick

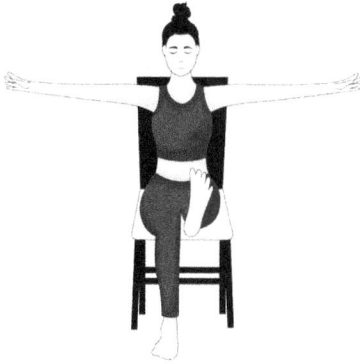

Sit up with the back straight.

Keep both your arms straight parallel to the floor at the shoulder level. Kick your left leg out slightly, pointing to the opposite corner, and then bring it back, but keep the arms at your side. Feel your core engaged. Alternate and continue for sixteen to twenty kicks.

Front Reach

Now energetically, keep reaching to the front, slightly angling at the opposite side. Keep alternating and counting a total of twenty moves.

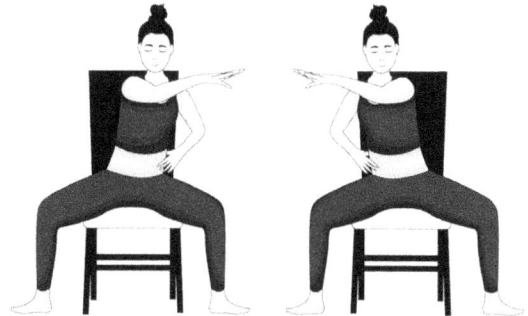

Front Punches

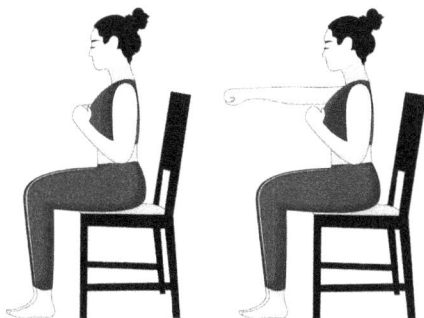

Keep your abdominals engaged. Bend your arms up so your wrists are by your shoulders. With control, slowly punch in front of, up, and across your body with one arm while slightly rotating your torso in the same direction. Return to the start position, then switch to the other arm. Alternate and repeat twenty times.

Overhead Punches

Bend your arms, and with control, slowly punch above your head with one arm. Fully straighten it, or as much as you can, and bring it down. Switch to the other arm. Alternate and repeat twenty times.

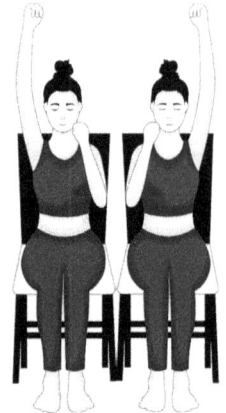

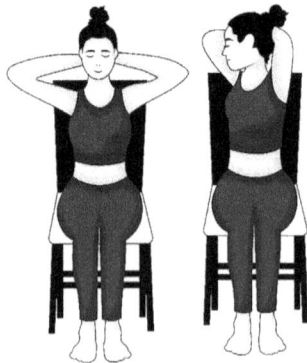

Torso Twist

Put your arms behind your head and keep your elbows wide. Feel your abdominals engaged, gently twist, return to the center, and turn on another side. Alternate and repeat ten to fourteen times.

Side Raise and Knee Raise

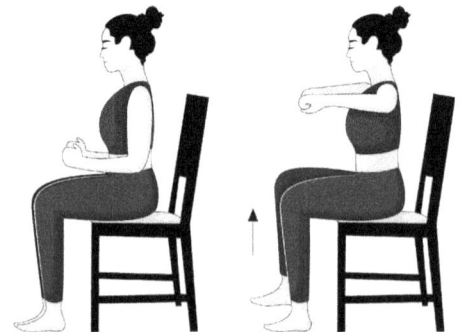

Keep both legs on the floor with knees bent at a 90-degree angle. Bend your elbows and lift them parallel to the floor at shoulder height. Simultaneously, lift one knee up. Bring the elbows and the knee back down. Repeat with the opposite knee—lift the elbows up with the opposite knee. Alternate and repeat twenty times. You can use weights for this movement.

Stand Up Flow

Keep your feet flat on the floor, shoulder-width apart, and underneath your hips. Keep your back and neck straight, with your chest slightly forward. Lean forward and slightly shift your weight to the front of your feet. Slowly stand up. Try not to support any weight with your hands. Take a full breath, and tighten your core and abdominal muscles to control your lowering as much as possible. Lower yourself to the chair with control. Repeat six to ten times.

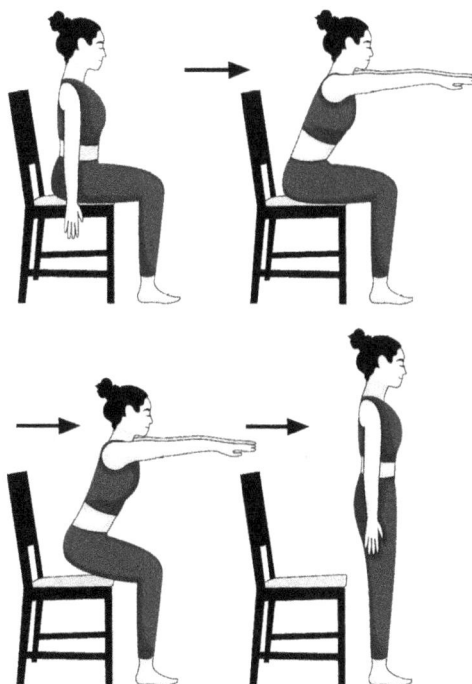

Seated Shoulder Press

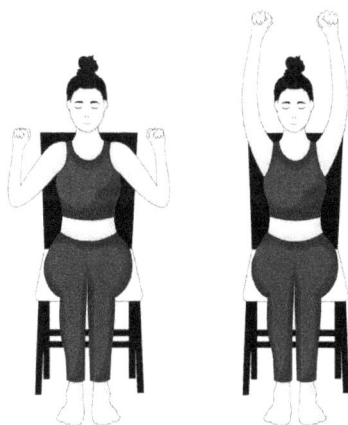

You can use weights if you want to, as this depends on your physical abilities. Using your body weight is also great for the workout. Engage the core muscles.

Begin with both elbows extended to the sides under the shoulders, chest lifted. Face forward with palms turned outward. Extend the arms upward, reaching above the head until fully extended or to a comfortable range. Avoid touching the hands together and keep both arms parallel. Gradually lower the hands to the starting position and maintain spread elbows. Avoid tucking the elbows toward the body's center; extend them outward until a gentle pinching sensation (not painful) is felt at the shoulder blades' top. Repeat eight to ten times.

DAY 24

Kick and Toe Touch

Take a short break if you need to. Keep the arms behind your head. Ensure you're not putting all the arm's weight and forcing your neck down. Keep your back straight and core engaged. Arms behind the head. Lift the leg and extend the opposite arm, trying to reach the toes of the opposite leg while the other arm stays behind the head. Alternate and repeat twelve to fourteen times.

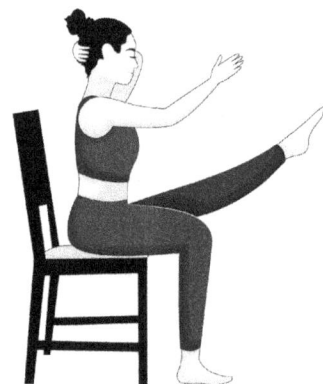

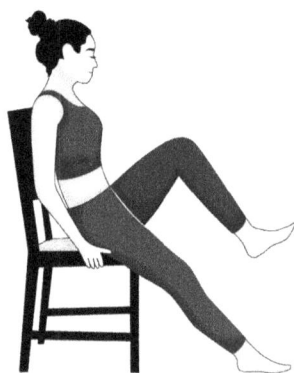

Bicycle Curls

Lean back into the chair and grab the edges of the chair. Extend one leg out and pull the knee back to your chest. Think if you're peddling the bicycle. Repeat on one side six to eight times. Switch to the opposite side. Now reverse—start with one leg peddling in the opposite direction. Switch sides and repeat six to eight times.

Flutter Kicks

Lean back into the chair with your spine straight. Fully extend your legs, hold the chair's edges, lift both legs.

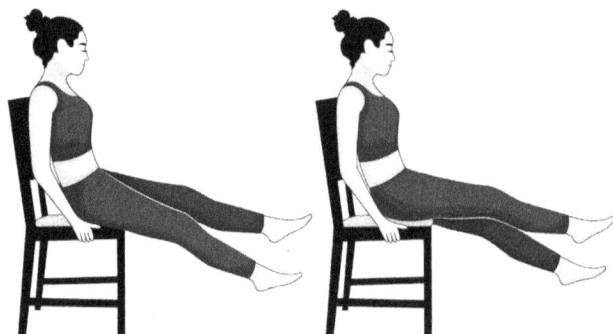

314

Single March with a Twist

Lean back into the chair with your back straight; don't round your back. Move the bottom toward the edge of the chair. You can hold the edges of the chair with your arms. Core engaged. Do single marches by lifting your knee as high as you can. Alternate and repeat ten to fourteen times.

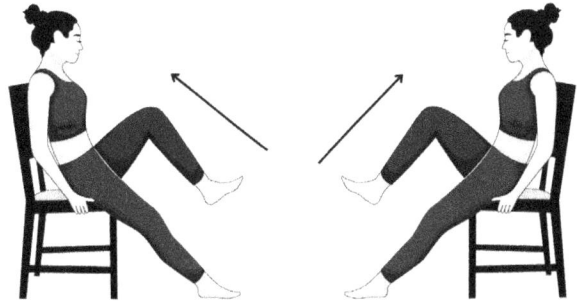

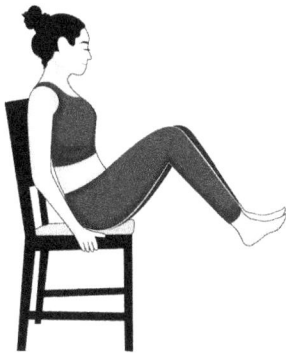

If you're feeling brave and strong, lift both knees simultaneously. Repeat six to eight times.

DAY 25

Modify Chair Squat

Start with your knees shoulder-width apart. Lean forward and lift your hips off the chair. If needed, you can hold the chair's edges for support as you safely return to the seated position. Alternatively, place your arms on your knees, but avoid leaning into them. Engage your glutes and hamstrings to assist in lifting your hips. Repeat this movement ten times.

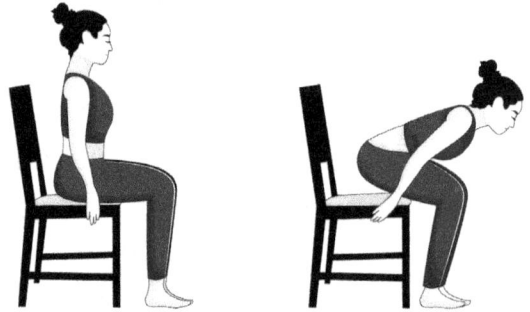

Straight Leg Raise Twist

Position yourself at the front of the chair. Extend your right leg while ensuring your left foot stays grounded. Cross your arms over your chest and engage your abdominal muscles. Rotate your torso to the right, lifting your right leg.

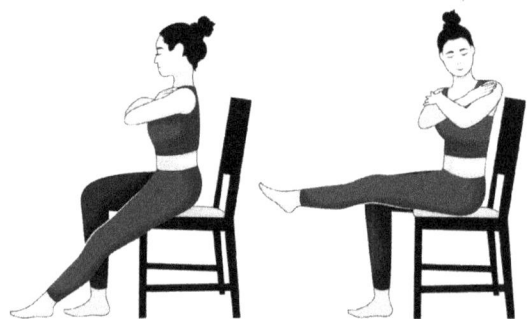

Squeeze your knees together and return to the starting position.

Switch sides and repeat. Alternate and repeat sixteen to twenty repetitions.

Seated Jacks with Straight Arms

Put the palms together with straight arms in front of you. Hold your knees together. Move closer to the front of the chair if you need to. Open your arms to the sides and step the right foot out to the sides. Open your hips as much as you can. Arms are returning to the middle, the same as the right foot. Alternate and repeat a total of twenty times.

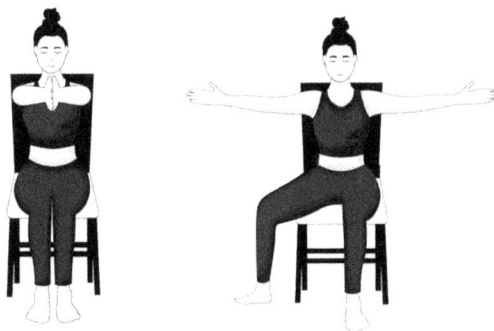

Lateral and Front Arm Raises

Ensure your back is straight. Engage your abs. Place your arms down by your sides. Slowly lift them with weight or without parallel to the ground at shoulder level. Slowly lower them down. Lift them in front of you—shoulder level and lower them down. Control the movement; don't swing your arms. Repeat eight to ten times. You can add weights.

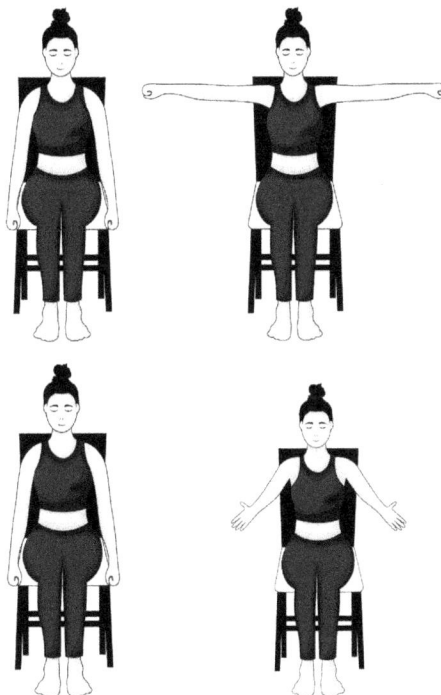

Seat Hollow body

Come to the front of the chair, and with your back straight, raise your arms. Lean back at about a 45-degree angle. You should feel a contraction in your abdominals. If it feels too much with your hands over your head, cross the arms on your chest and hold. Focus on your abs. Maintain the back straight and keep leaning back.

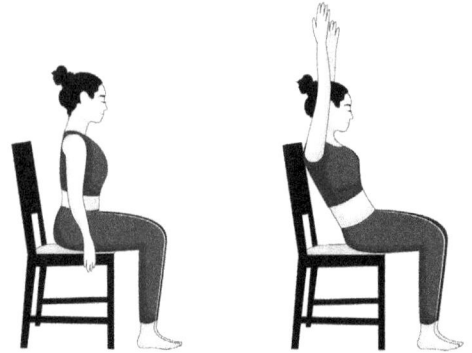

Slowly count to 30. Take a few breaths, rest, and repeat it.

Elbow to Knee

Keep feet flat on the floor and shoulders rolled back. Feel your abs engaged. Place your hands behind your head, elbows pointing out to the sides. Lift your right knee toward your chest while simultaneously bringing the left elbow toward your right knee. Return to the starting position with control. Repeat on the opposite side. Alternate and repeat eight to ten times.

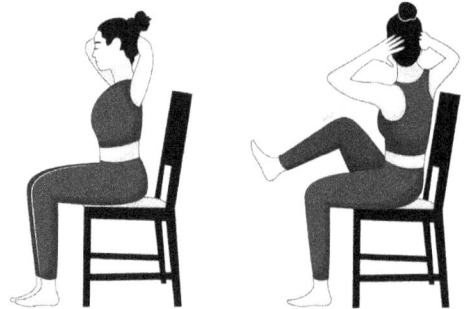

Seated Jacks

Move closer to the front of the chair with arms at your sides. In a harmonious motion, lift your arms overhead, fingertips gently meeting, with palms turned outward. Simultaneously, extend both legs out as your arms ascend. Bring both legs back to the center as your arms land. Repeat eight to ten times.

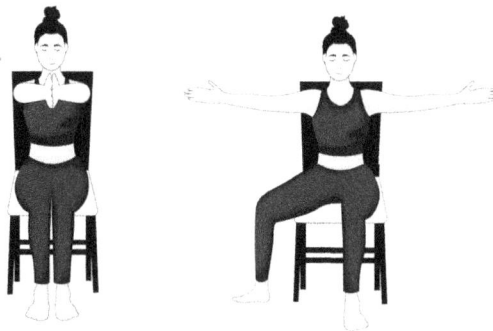

If extending both legs and arms simultaneously is too challenging, try this version instead.

Observe your breathing and body. Do it at a pace that suits you.

Try not to hold your breath.

Skater Switch

Shift to the front of your chair.

Bend your right knee while extending your left leg to the opposite side.

Keep your toes pointed.

Start extending your arms. Lean forward and attempt to reach the inside of your right foot with your left arm. Swiftly switch and repeat the movement with the right arm and the left foot. The back is straight. Alternate sides and repeat twenty-five to thirty times.

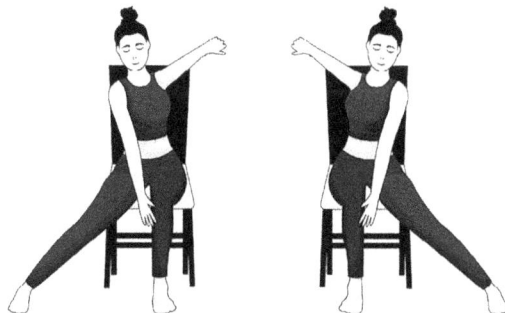

DAY 26

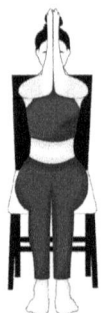 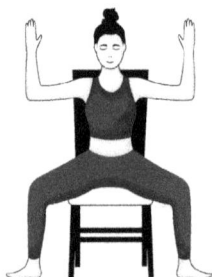

Hips Opener

Open both arms and hips to sides simultaneously. Repeat five to eight times.

Leg and Opposite Arm Raise

Inhale and raise the right leg and left arm. Hold for a few breaths.

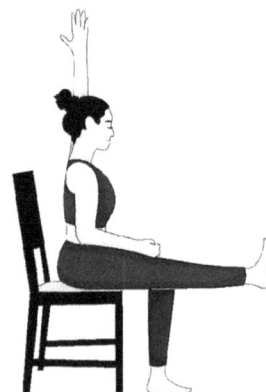

Feel how your leg is activated. Lower the leg or bend through the knee if it's too challenging. Release to the ground after a couple of breaths. Repeat two to three times for each side.

Chair Squats

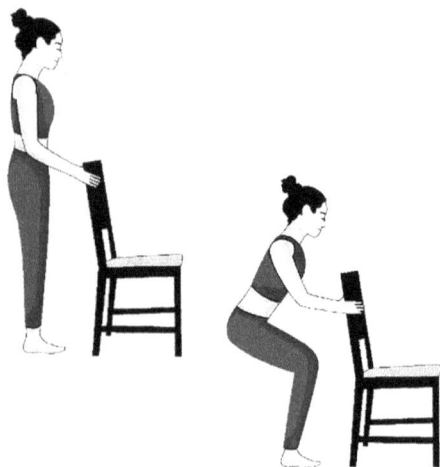

Stand at the back of the chair, holding onto the sides of the chair if help with balance is needed. Inhale, stand tall, grounding down into the soles of the feet, extending the spine upward. Exhale and sit weight back into heels. If you need a bigger challenge—your toes can be lifted to exaggerate the weight in the heels. Lower belly pulled in. The knees should be positioned behind the toes. Keep length in the spine and the back of the neck. Hold for three breaths. Repeat three times.

Shoulder Stretch

Bring your hands behind the head. Pull your elbows back as much as possible; imagine your shoulder blades having to keep a pencil between them. And then slowly move your elbows forward, trying to touch each other. Repeat the movement three to five times.

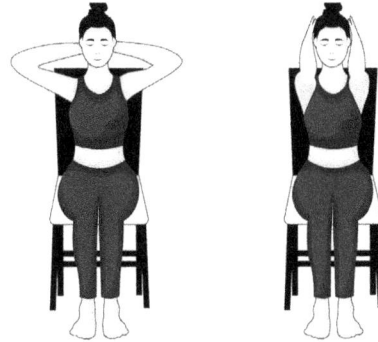

Lateral Arm Raises

Raise your arms parallel to the ground and at shoulder height, and lower them back to your sides. Feel your abdominal wall engaged, and don't hinge in the shoulders. Repeat the movement eight to ten times.

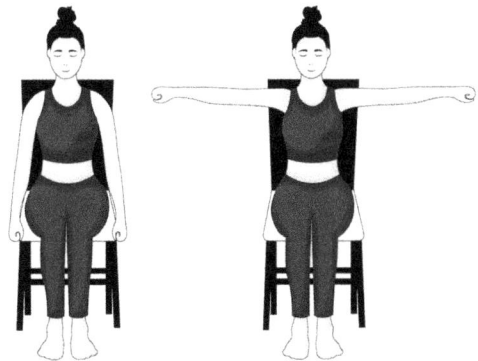

Plank Pose with Chair

Place your hands on the seat of the chair. Stack shoulders over hands, walk your feet back, hip-distance apart. Depending on your body's abilities, walk your feet as far as you feel comfortable. You can be on your toes or feet flat, core engaged. Observe your shoulders being stacked over your wrists. Keep your spine straight. Long line from shoulders to feet. Hold five long, deep breaths or less.

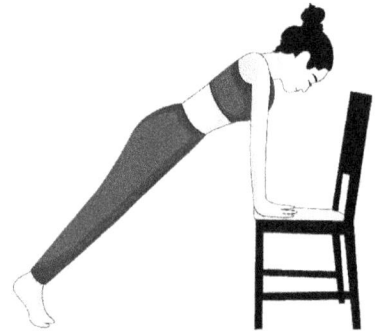

DAY 27

Elegant Kick

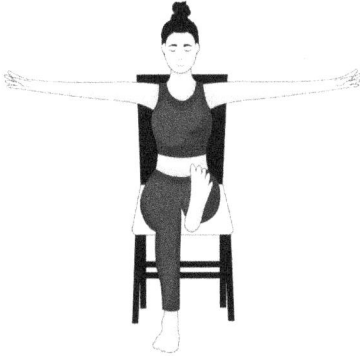

Sit up with the back straight.

Keep both your arms straight parallel to the floor at the shoulder level. Kick your left leg out slightly, pointing to the opposite corner, and then bring it back, but keep the arms at your side. Feel your core engaged. Alternate and continue for sixteen to twenty kicks.

Knee to Nose

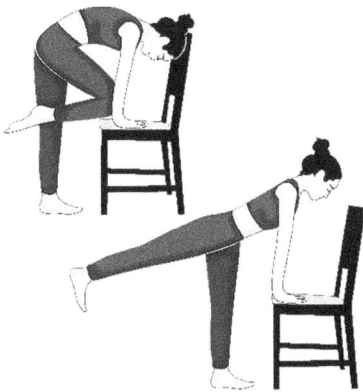

Begin by standing tall and upright, squarely facing the chair seat. Place your hands on the chair. Glide your right leg behind you to its fullest extent. As you exhale, draw the right knee toward your nose, curving it inward. Inhale again, send the leg back by extending it, creating length, and then exhale to bring the knee toward your nose again. Repeat this fluid sequence a total of six to ten times on one side. Mirror the sequence on the opposite side, maintaining your focus and intention throughout.

One Leg Backlit

Keep your hands on the back of the chair. Stand tall. Bring your weight to the right foot. Extend the left leg back and lift off the ground. The toes of both feet are pointing forward. Move back and forth six to ten times. Repeat with the opposite leg. Repeat twice on each side.

Chair Pose Above Chair

Maintain an upright posture and lift your arms above your head while exhaling deeply. Inhale and move into a chair pose, gently raising yourself to your feet above the chair. Exhale and return to a seated position, arms still extended overhead. Inhale again and resume the chair pose. Repeat this sequence six times to ten times.

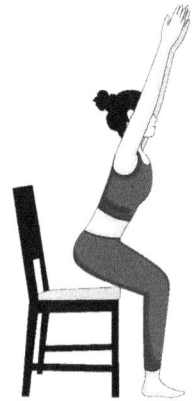

Step and Press

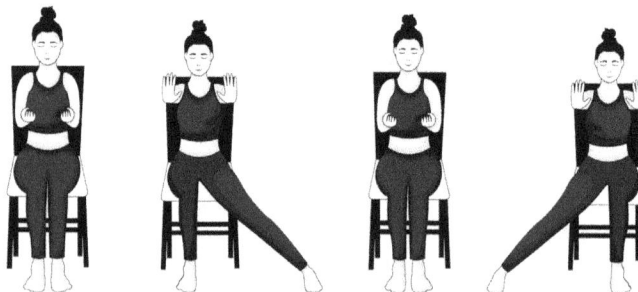

Keep your back straight, and keep the elbows bent with your palm facing out. Make a 90-degree angle on both sides (cactus arms). Press it up, and at the same time, step one foot to the side and keep your knee slightly bent. Pull your arms back and step the leg back to the center. Alternate and repeat twenty times

DAY 28

Shoulder Rolls

Start by bringing your shoulder to your ears. Slowly and gently roll them back and then forward. Repeat ten times.

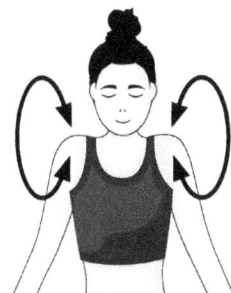

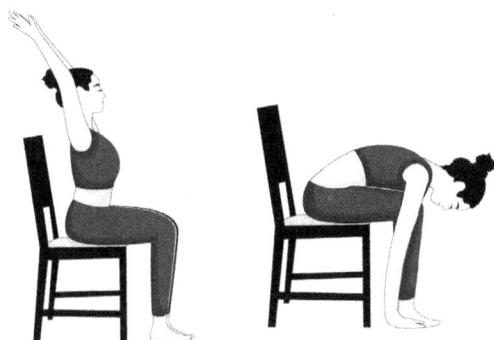

Forward Fold

On the inhale, raise your arms up and gently stretch. On the exhale, take the arms toward your feet, with the torso resting on the thighs and chin close to the knees. Feel a stretch across your shoulders and back. To release, inhale, look up first, then raise your arms before returning to sit. Remain in the pose for two breaths or till you feel comfortable.

Side Stretches

Raise your arms overhead. Extend away from the floor, maintaining open elbows. Inhale gently, drawing your shoulder blades slightly back. Engage your core and bend to the right from your torso. Exhale and switch sides. Alternate and repeat eight to ten times.

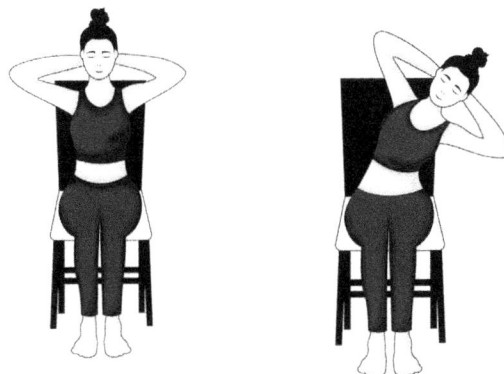

Hamstring Stretch

Sit closer to the front of the chair. Extend one leg in front of you, pulling the toes toward you. Lean as far as you can. Feel the hamstring stretch. Remain for two to three breaths. Switch the legs.

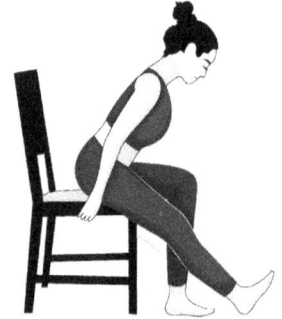

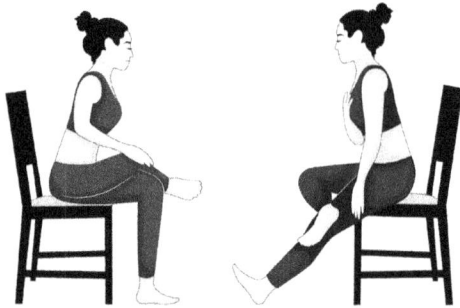

Seated Figure Four or Pigeon Pose

Put your right ankle over the left knee or on the left shin. With your back straight, lean forward and remain for a few breaths, feeling the stretch in your hip. Repeat on the other side.

Upper Body Twist

Engage your core. Keep the chin slightly tucked in. Cross your arms on your chest and twist to the right. Return to the center and then twist to the left. Alternate and repeat six to eight times.

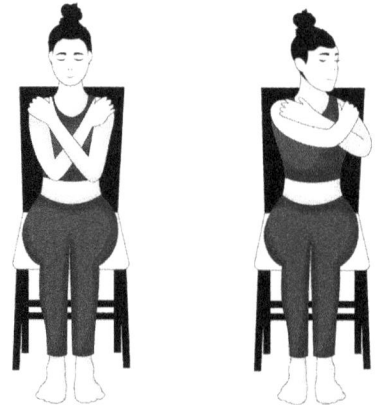

Cat-Cow Position

Place your arms on your knees. As you inhale, expand your chest, allowing your head and chin to tilt slightly back. On the exhale, round your spine by curling your chest inward. Ensure your shoulders are relaxed, and be aware of the space between your shoulders and earlobes.

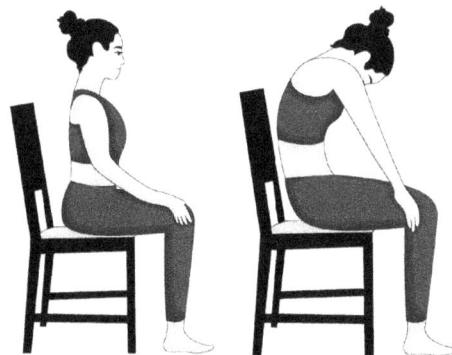

Practice coordinating your breath with the movement, moving at a comfortable pace. Repeat five to eight times.

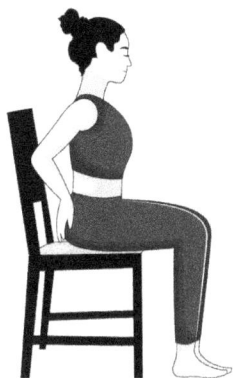

Back Stretch

Move closer to the edge of the chair. Put your palms on your lower back and pull your elbows and shoulders back. Feel your ribcage coming forward. Remain in the position for about thirty seconds.

Conclusion

It is exercise alone that supports the spirits,
and keeps the mind in vigor.

— Marcus Tullius Cicero

Who would have thought that a chair could be a starting block and the finish line in the grand marathon of life, where every sprint, stumble, and snack break count?

This book has sought to guide you on your journey to physical wellness—from finding your why and starting with the combination of healthy eating and exercising to staying motivated. It should be noted in closing that this journey you are on is ever-evolving, and there is no end point, per se.

I've learned that wellness isn't a destination; it's a constantly changing landscape. It's like playing a game of tag with your former self—just when you think you've caught up, there's another version of you, slightly healthier, waving from the horizon.

So, to you, dear reader, embarking on this *chair-ful* journey to a fitter self, remember: it's a path strewn with laughter, the occasional tear, and maybe a few too many protein bars. One day, you'll look back at this version of yourself and chuckle at the memory of thinking, "How hard can exercising with a chair be?"

Embrace the journey, the chair, and maybe even the occasional indulgence. After all, what's life without a little extra seasoning? Here's to finding your balance—both on the chair and in life.

Take a seat, and happy exercising!

You Could Be Key to Someone Else's Yoga Journey

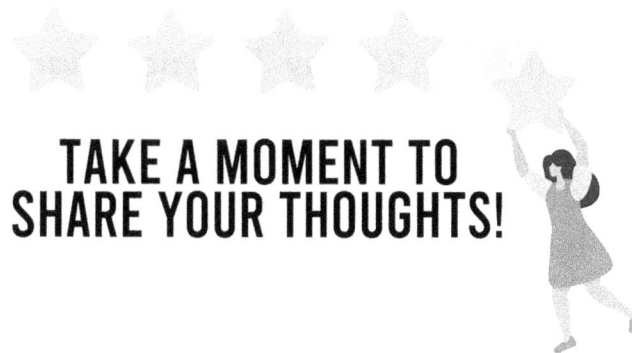

TAKE A MOMENT TO SHARE YOUR THOUGHTS!

Thank you so much for your support. No matter what might hold us back from standing yoga, we can still access its astounding potential... And with your help, I can make sure that the message reaches even more people.

Check Out More Books by Ottie Oz

If you enjoyed this book, you might also find these titles by Ottie Oz interesting and helpful:

Transform Your Balance: A 28-Day Exercise Plan for Seniors

Improve your stability and confidence with exercises specifically designed for seniors looking to address balance issues or better their skills. Our program includes targeted activities such as standing on one leg and walking heel-to-toe, ensuring each exercise effectively supports your balance. Follow along with our clear, silent video demonstrations for each exercise.

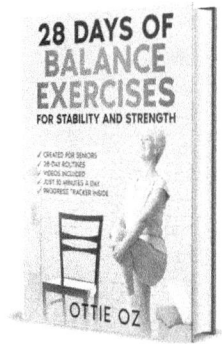

Transform Your Life: Manage Your Knee Pain

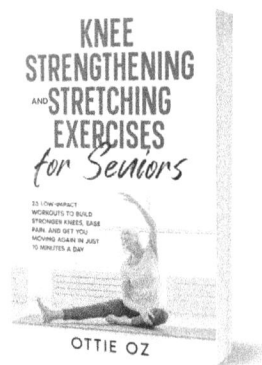

Discover how to manage and reduce knee pain with our effective guide, designed to strengthen and mobilize your knees in just 10 minutes a day. Improve your walking, enhance flexibility, and regain confidence to engage in your favorite activities with less discomfort. Our book offers simple, step-by-step exercises with clear illustrations, suitable for doing at home without any special equipment

Kickstart your journey to a stronger, healthier you with our 28-day chair exercise program.

It's designed for anyone looking to enhance their overall health. Perfect for those recovering from knee surgery, managing limited mobility, or juggling a busy schedule, this guide offers gentle yet effective exercises tailored to your needs.

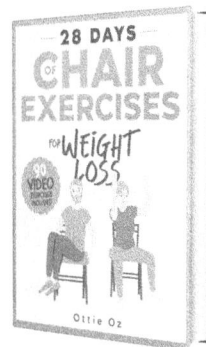

Inside, you'll find 99 easy exercises illustrated with clear pictures and simple instructions, ideal for both beginners and intermediates to progress at their own pace. All video demonstrations are now hosted on YouTube for easy access, ensuring you can follow along with proper form to feel confident, avoid injuries, and get the most out of your workouts. Alongside physical exercise, the book includes healthy eating tips to support gradual, sustainable weight loss and nourish your body with balanced habits.

Designed for everyone, no matter your age or ability, this program aims to make fitness accessible and achievable.

Start Your 28-Day Chair Yoga Challenge

Struggling with joint pain, limited movement, or a fear of falling? Discover the 28-Day Chair Yoga Challenge. This guide offers a straightforward approach to feeling better and moving easier, with exercises you can perform from a chair. Each day presents a new routine, enhancing your strength and flexibility without standing up.

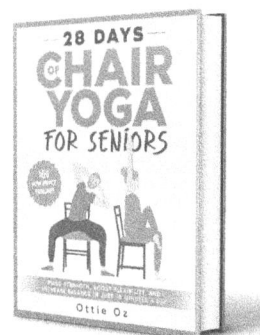

This book provides over 180 pictures to guide you through each exercise, complemented by video demonstrations on YouTube. Spend just 10 minutes a day to improve your health and regain independence in your daily activities.

Embrace a pain-free lifestyle with routines that build muscle, enhance mobility, and boost confidence—all from the safety and comfort of your chair.

Visit Ottie Oz's Author Page for more information and to discover other great books.

References

Admin-Calimobility. (2023, April 13). 21 Chair Exercises for Seniors: Complete visual guide. California Mobility. https://californiamobility. com/21-chair-exercises-for-seniors-visual-guide/.

Ascm-Cep, L. W. M. (2022, October 1). 11 chair exercises for seniors. Verywell Fit. https://www.verywellfit.com/chair-exercises-for-seniors-4161267.

A-Z Quotes. (n.d.). *Marcus Tullius Cicero quote*. https://www.azquotes. com/quote/566618.

BrainyQuote. (n.d.). *Friedrich Nietzsche quotes*. https://www. brainyquote.com/quotes/friedrich_nietzsche_103819.

Callahan, A., Leonard, H., & Powell, T. (2020). *Nutrition in adults*. Open Oregon Educational Resources. https://openoregon.pressbooks. pub/nutritionscience/chapter/11f-older-adults/.

Carter, C. (2012, January 2). *Please quit your diet, now*. Greater Good. https://greatergood.berkeley.edu/article/item/Quit_Diet_Now.

Centers for Disease Control and Prevention. (2019). *How much physical activity do older adults need?* https://www.cdc.gov/physicalactivity/ basics/older_adults/index.htm.

Centers for Disease Control and Prevention. (2022, September 19). *Losing weight*. https://www.cdc.gov/healthyweight/losing_weight/ index.html.

Coratella, G., Tornatore, G., Longo, S., Esposito, F., & Cè, E. (2020). *An electromyographic analysis of lateral raise variations and frontal raise in competitive bodybuilders. International Journal of Environmental Research and Public Health*, *17*(17) , 6015. https://doi.org/10.3390/ijerph17176015.

Cscs, I. L. M. (2018, September 28). Seated Flexibility, Cardio, & Strength Workout. EatingWell. https://www.eatingwell.com/article/290859/seated-flexibility-cardio-strength-workout/.

Dattani, S., Ortiz-Ospina, E., Ritchie, H., Rodés-Guirao, L., & Roser, M. (2023). *Life expectancy*. Our World in Data. https://ourworldindata.org/life-expectancy.

Fitness Expo. (n.d.). How to lose weight while sitting at the office. https://www.fitnessexpostores.com/how-to-lose-weight-while-sitting-at-the-office/.

Greatist. (n.d.). Chair exercises. https://greatist.com/fitness/chair-exercises#sit-to-stands.

Goodreads. (n.d.). *A quote by Edward Stanley*. https://www.goodreads.com/quotes/173133-those-who-think-they-have-not-time-for-bodily-exercise.

Greenberg, M. (2013, May 21). *The best quotes on healthy living*. Psychology Today. https://www.psychologytoday.com/intl/blog/the-mindful-self-express/201305/the-best-quotes-healthy-living.

King, A. C. (2001). Interventions to promote physical activity by older adults. The Journals of Gerontology: Series A, 56(Supplement 2) , 36–46. https://doi.org/10.1093/gerona/56.suppl_2.36.

Laird, E., Rasmussen, C. L., Kenny, R. A., & Herring, M. P. (2023). Physical activity dose and depression in a cohort of older adults in the Irish Longitudinal Study on Ageing. *JAMA Network*, *6*(7). https://doi.org/10.1001/jamanetworkopen.2023.22489.

Lalanne, J. (n.d.). *Quotes — Jack Lalanne*. Jack Lalanne. https://jacklalanne.com/quotes/.

Louw, S., Makwela, S., Manas, L., Meyer, L., Terblanche, D., & Brink, Y. (2017). Effectiveness of exercise in office workers with neck pain: A systematic review and meta-analysis. *South African Journal of Physiotherapy*, *73*(1). https://doi.org/10.4102/sajp.v73i1.392.

Mann, T., Tomiyama, A. J., Westling, E., Lew, A.-M., Samuels, B., & Chatman, J. (2007). Medicare's search for effective obesity treatments: Diets are not the answer. *American Psychologist*, *62*(3) , 220–233. https://doi.org/10.1037/0003-066x.62.3.220.

Mayo Clinic. (2023, September 21). *How do exercise and arthritis fit together?* https://www.mayoclinic.org/diseases-conditions/arthritis/in-depth/arthritis/art-20047971.

National Health Service. (2021, November 4). *Understanding calories*. https://www.nhs.uk/live-well/healthy-weight/managing-your-weight/understanding-calories/.

O'Toole, G. O. (2021, August 24). *How old would you be if you didn't know how old you are?* Quote Investigator. https://quoteinvestigator.com/2021/08/24/how-old/.

Picorelli, A. M. A., Pereira, L. S. M., Pereira, D. S., Felício, D., & Sherrington, C. (2014). Adherence to exercise programs for older people is influenced by program characteristics and personal factors: a systematic review. *Journal of Physiotherapy*, *60*(3) , 151–156. https://doi.org/10.1016/j.jphys.2014.06.012.

Quote Investigator. (2019, April 18). *Take the first step in faith.* https://quoteinvestigator.com/2019/04/18/staircase/.

Seated exercise. (n.d.). https://www.active-charnwood.org/seated-exercise.

Slater, D. (2020, May 10). Lower and upper limb exercises. Keheren Therapy. https://www.keherentherapy.co.uk/chair-exercises-seniors/.

Smith, J. (2021, April 10). 5 Exercise Myths for People 55 and Older. Impact Physical Therapy. https://impactpthillsboro.com/5-exercise-myths-for-people-55-and-older/.

Smith, J. (2013, May 6). 6 seated moves that work your whole body. Shape. https://www.shape.com/fitness/workouts/6-seated-moves-work-your-whole-body.

Times of India. (n.d.). Burn the FUPA: 5 seated chair poses to get rid of lower belly fat. https://timesofindia.indiatimes.com/life-style/health-fitness/weight-loss/burn-the-fupa-5-seated-chair-poses-to-get-rid-of-lower-belly-fat/photostory/95213618.cms?picid=95213633.

U.S. Department of Health and Human Services. (2018). *Physical activity guidelines for Americans 2nd edition* (p. 32). https://health.gov/sites/default/files/2019-09/Physical_Activity_Guidelines_2nd_edition.pdf#page=32.

United Nations, Department of Economic and Social Affairs, Population Division (2022). *World Population Prospects 2022, Online Edition.* https://population.un.org/wpp/Download/Standard/Population/.

USDA. (2020). *Dietary guidelines for Americans 2020-2025.* https://www.dietaryguidelines.gov/sites/default/files/2021-03/Dietary_Guidelines_for_Americans-2020-2025.pdf.

Vive Health. (n.d.). 22 Chair exercises for Seniors & How to get started. https://www.vivehealth.com/blogs/resources/chair-exercises-for-seniors.

Website, N. (2022b, June 13). Sitting exercises. nhs.uk. https://www.nhs.uk/live-well/exercise/strength-and-flexibility-exercises/sitting-exercises/.

Wilson, C. H. (1927). [Newspaper]. Sermon.

World Health Organization. (2018). *Typhoid vaccines: WHO position paper, March 2018 — Recommendations. Vaccine, 37*(2). https://doi.org/10.1016/j.vaccine.2018.04.022.

World Health Organization. (2020, December 9). *The top 10 causes of death.* https://www.who.int/news-.

www.ingramcontent.com/pod-product-compliance
Lightning Source LLC
Chambersburg PA
CBHW080605270326
41928CB00016B/2928

9781916947153